Edgar Cayce (
Health, Healing, and Rejuvenation

John Van Auken

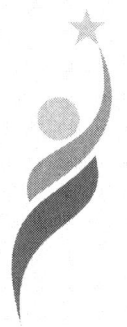

Living in the Light
Virginia Beach, Virginia USA

ISBN-13: 978-1532723490
ISBN-10: 1532723490

JohnVanAuken.com
JohnVanAuken.Newsletter@Gmail.com

Living in the Light
P.O. Box 4942
Virginia Beach VA 23454 USA

Other books by this author
are available from
Amazon.com
Createspace.com
AREcatalog.com
JohnVanAuken.com

John Van Auken is the Director of the
Edgar Cayce Foundation

CONTENTS

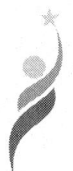

List of Illustrations

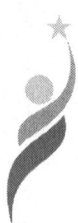

—Disclaimer—

Nothing I wrote in this book should replace cooperating with educated, licensed healthcare practitioners. Self diagnosis and prescription by only reading health material is not a good approach to health. Learn all you can but then consult with licensed healthcare professionals. These people have spent years in education and study; many have years of experience with human health. What you find in this book to be helpful should be used in cooperation with an educated, licensed healthcare practitioner.

–John Van Auken

—About the References in this Book—

Throughout this book you will see references in parentheses of a number followed by another number, like this: (262-26). These refer to the specific location of this material within the volumes of the Edgar Cayce files. The first number replaces the name of the person or persons seeking the information in an effort to provide some privacy. The second number identifies the sequence in their specific series of discourses. In my example, 262 is the number for a group of persons seeking spiritual information, and -26 reveals that this is the 26th discourse in the 262's series of questioning Cayce.

Also, when Cayce raised his voice for emphasis his stenographer put those words in capital LETTERS. When you see capitalized words in the middle of a sentence know that he intended to put emphasis on that word. Normally today we would *italicize* such words but she capitalized them.

His discourses are often referred to as "readings," because it felt as if he were "reading" a person's mind, body, and soul, or their "Book of Life" or Akashic Record.

The readings are available on CD-ROM, in printed books, online at the Cayce website, and in the files at the Edgar Cayce Center. The Center is located on the roughly 5-acre campus of the Association for Research and Enlightenment at 215 67th Street in Virginia Beach, Virginia, 23451, U.S.A. The website is EdgarCayce.org. The central phone number is 757-428-3588 or toll free 800-333-4499.

About Edgar Cayce

In 1979, the *Journal of the American Medical Association*
credited Edgar Cayce with initiating
the American holistic health movement.
–JAMA 1979:241(11):1156.

Most every day for over forty years of his adult life, Edgar Cayce would lie down on a couch with his hands folded over his stomach and allow himself to enter a self-induced hypnotic/meditative state. Then, when provided with the name and location of an individual anywhere in the world he would speak in a normal voice and give answers to any questions about that person or their life in general. Questions as diverse as, "How can I remove a wart?" and "What are the secrets of the universe?" were asked. His responses to these questions came to be called "readings" and contain insights so valuable that even to this day individuals rely upon them as practical help for maintaining a well-balanced diet, improving human relationships, and overcoming life-threatening illnesses – including such far-reaching inquiries about the origin and destiny of the body, mind, and soul!

These "readings" were written down by a stenographer, who kept one copy on file and sent another to the person or persons who had requested the information. Much of this information was given from the 1920s through the 1940s. Subsequent to this time period many have added and update new findings and research reports and are a part of the body of work maintained by the Edgar Cayce Center.

Edgar Cayce never wrote a book. But many books have been written about him. And though Cayce died nearly a century ago, the timeliness of the material is evidenced by approximately a dozen biographies and more than 300 titles that discuss various aspects of this man's life and work. Further details about his life and work are explored in such classic works as *There Is a River* (1942) by Thomas Sugrue, *The Sleeping Prophet* (1967) by bestselling author Jess Stearn, *Many Mansions* (1950) by Gina Cerminara, and *Edgar Cayce: An American Prophet* (2000) by Sidney Kirkpatrick.

Words that are fairly common in today's lexicon, such as meditation, auras, soul mates, and holism derive from Edgar Cayce and his readings.

I have read most of the readings and much about Cayce. And I have had the good fortune to have lived and worked with his sons, many of the people who received readings from Cayce, and many of the early supporters and employees of the organization. And I have incorporated his advice into my personal life.

Cayce was a fascinating man. He was born on March 18, 1877, and reared in the small community of Hopkinsville, Kentucky. He quit school after eight years to work on the family farm. Eventually Cayce took up photography as his trade.

In addition to being a devout member of the local churches wherever he was living, Cayce faithfully taught Sunday School and held to the basic tenets of Christianity. He even entertained the thought of becoming a minister, but his lack of education and finances forced him to turn in another direction.

Indeed, in the early years of his "readings" he found himself concerned about possible conflicts between his religious beliefs, the teachings of the church, and the phenomenon that he was experiencing. In time, he came to feel that his gift was a manifestation of God's will and reinforced, rather than ruptured, his religious beliefs. Because of this acceptance, he continued with his readings. He would give over 14,000 readings during his adult lifetime.

Under the influence of a self-induced hypnotic-like trance, Cayce would diagnose illnesses and suggest treatments ailing individuals.

During a trance he would often use long medical terms that were normally used only by physicians. Upon awakening, he could hardly pronounce the words much less understand their meanings.

Edgar Cayce's first spiritual encounter occurred when he was only a toddler. He often spoke of "invisible playmates" who would visit him, (Thomas Sugrue, *There Is A River*, p. 37). He also claimed to have a visitation from a "shining lady" who said he could have anything he desired. He responded that he would like to help people, especially children (p. 23). On one occasion, when he was having trouble studying his school lessons, this "shining lady" told him to lay his head on the textbook and rest. He obeyed and quickly fell asleep. After a few minutes he returned to consciousness and knew the entire content of the volume, (p. 19).

At the age of 20, Cayce mysteriously lost his voice. He consulted several doctors, took numerous prescriptions, and finally resorted to home remedies. But nothing worked.

A traveling hypnotist attempted to cure the malady, but failed. A friend, Al Layne, suggested that Edgar undertake an effort of self-hypnosis, whereby he could diagnose his own illness and prescribe a cure. The experiment was successful! (pp. 121-122)

Cayce lost his voice on several other occasions. Each time he would slip into a trace and get a "reading" on himself and cure the problem. Layne was ecstatic. He encouraged his friend to go into business as a trance medium. Convinced that he could help others with so-called incurable ailments, Cayce began scheduling readings.

Edgar Cayce's fame spread. On October 9, 1910, an issue of the *New York Times'* headlined declared, "Illiterate Man Becomes a Doctor When Hypnotized. Strange Power Shown By Edgar Cayce Puzzles Physicians." The article piqued the interest of its readers and within weeks thousands of letters poured into Hopkinsville from people seeking medical help.

For twenty years the so-called "sleeping prophet" offered help to those in need.

But the use of his extra-sensory powers would soon be altered when Art Lammers, a wealthy printer and student of metaphysics, approached Cayce for a reading. Lammers was not concerned about health, however; he wanted to know about the future. He wanted a "life reading!" Lammers drilled the unconscious medium about the end of the world, creation, the lost continent of Atlantis, the path of salvation and a host of other religious-type subjects, (p. 234). Cayce responded. He proclaimed the world to be a pantheistic manifestation of God, announced that reincarnation was the secret of ultimate reconciliation of man to God and that Jesus became the first perfected man by being reincarnated some thirty times! Though these revelations flew against the teachings of his church, Edgar Cayce eventually accepted the discourse as true.

Others sought life readings (as apposed to health readings). Some wanted to make contact with the spirits of soldiers who had been killed during World War I or II. The spirits manifested themselves through Cayce's vocal cords. They brought messages of hope and assurance that Heaven awaits mankind. His life readings not only looked into the past but into the future. In history, for example, the Cayce readings gave insights into Essene Judaism that were verified a decade *after* his death. In world affairs, he saw the collapse of communism nearly fifty years *before* it happened. He spoke of legendary Troy as though it was truly an ancient city, long before its ruins were discovered in Turkey. Repeatedly, science and history have validated concepts and ideas explored in Cayce's psychic information.

In the field of psychology, he has often been compared to Carl Jung. In the realm of education, he stands with Rudolf Steiner. Dr. Richard H. Drummond, one of the world's most renowned theological scholars, called the Cayce information on spirituality "the finest devotional material of the 20th century."

There was a time when mainstream healthcare in the United States did not recognize any connections between a person's body, mind, and spirit. Today, holistic health is mainstream!

In 1931, Cayce and his family, and a band of his supporters founded the Association for Research and Enlightenment (A.R.E.) to be a depository for his readings. Each reading was categorized and filed for future reference. The headquarters are located on roughly five acres in Virginia Beach, Virginia. The Center operates a 50,000-volume library of metaphysics, houses an extensive research on metaphysics, health, and history. On the campus today are a holistic health center and spa, an accredited university with a Master's Degree in Transpersonal Psychology and Leadership, and a conference center offering lectures on a daily basis. Visitors are welcome. The Edgar Cayce web site has become so popular that it receives some 100,000 visitors *each month!* That's more than Edgar Cayce saw in his entire life. Online courses are available as well as a huge health database. The web site is EdgarCayce.org. In addition to the web site events and seminars are occurring around the world through a network of outreach programs.

The Edgar Cayce Center keeps the memory and work of Edgar Cayce alive and expanding. Copies of more than 14,000 of Edgar Cayce's readings are available to the public and have been filed along with any follow-up reports. This material represents the most massive collection of psychic information ever obtained from a single source.

—by Lyle E. Davis and John Van Auken

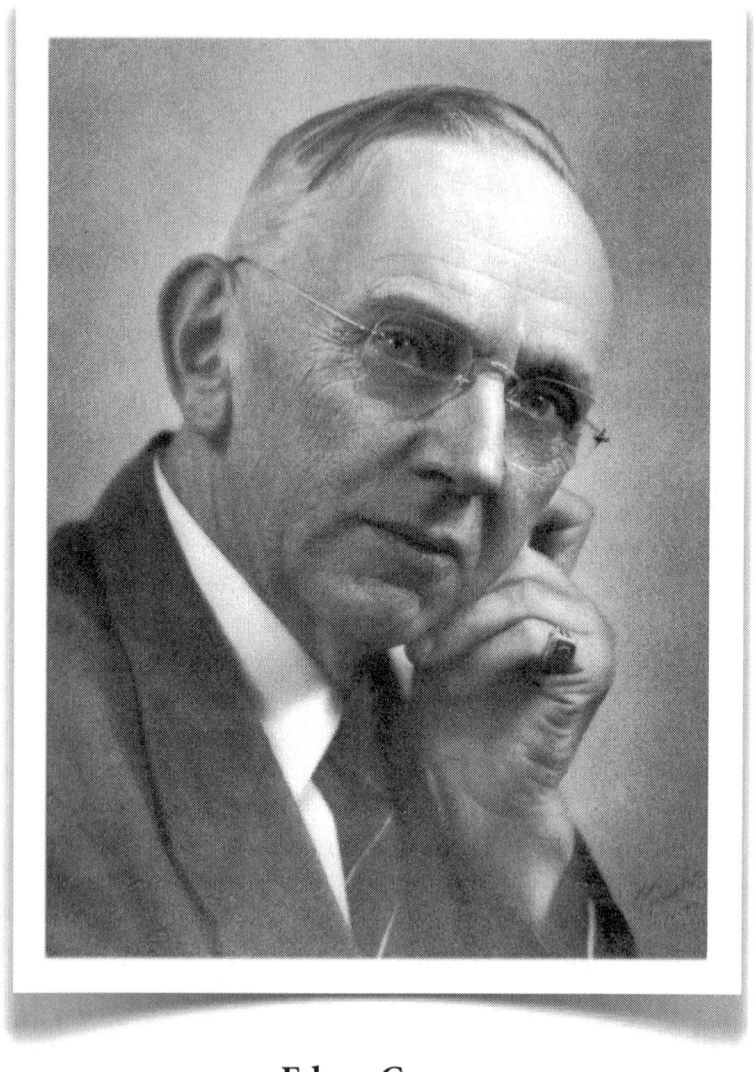

Edgar Cayce

Edgar Cayce's last name is the French version of the English
name *Casey*, and is pronounced the same, *kay-see*.

Foreword
Experiences with these Concepts

What you are about to read contains some of the finest concepts, methods, insights, and approaches to health, healing, and rejuvenation available for nearly 100 years – longer if we consider the ancient origins of holistic healing. I mean this sincerely and have seen the positive effects on living people that I've known including myself.

However, I have also witnessed these remedies and practices *not* working. Why? That is the question that challenges all of us to answer. Over many years I have interviewed professional healthcare people (MDs, nurses, and licensed practitioners), each having had much experience applying the Cayce health methods. Most every one of them shared their successes and failures. Almost to a person these professionals shared with me that the same approach for the same ailment that has worked on so many *does not work for everyone.* Their conclusion is that healing, that is, *real recovery* from degeneration or serious illness depends on some factor or factors associated with *the individual* seeking improvement.

Therefore, you must proceed with an attitude of testing, observation, and evaluation of each concept, method, ingredient, and activity given in this book. Be honest with yourself and your body and those you may be striving to help. But you must also be aware that a doubting mind and attitude will inhibit anything you're trying. I realize how paradoxical this is – I have lived with that paradox myself. But I also know firsthand that understanding the condition and treatment needed to maintain, heal, and renew the body can only become clear by pursuing the effort honestly, objectively, with hope and expectancy. The Edgar Cayce readings encourage testing these ideas personally and deciding for yourself if they are helpful.

And do not ignore our highly educated, licensed healthcare practitioners in a *cooperative* course of action. They have not only spent years of education and training but have passed often stringent licensing tests and requirements. And many of them have years of experience with patients having different conditions and circumstances. Many are open to cooperating in our endeavor to be healthy. Yes, they do have set protocols (official procedures and rules) that they must work within, and lawyers hold them responsible to these set protocols. But as long as you are not doing something they know to be harmful, they will usually cooperate with you in your holistic efforts.

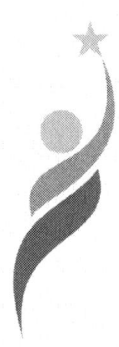

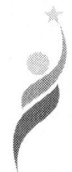

Chapter 1
WHY LIVE?

I suppose at sometime or another every soul must ask themselves this question. And it is a question to which we have a good answer, so before we seek our health, healing, and rejuvenation, let's explore this rather heavy question.

According to Edgar Cayce's channeled wisdom this incarnation is intentional and it is an important *opportunity* for our souls. Cayce's readings encourage us to "keep the physical fit, the soul will never die. Keep the physical fit that the soul may manifest the longer." (294-7) He gives two reasons, (1) Keep the physical fit for through the physical other physical beings benefit from our presence in their lives. This is the theme of the popular old movie *It's a Wonderful Life*, starring Jimmy Stewart and Donna Reed. Life without us would be much different for our friends, family, coworkers, and those we meet casually over the course of a lifetime. Our presence adds to the lives of others. And when our *better* selves are more often expressed our presence enhances their lives!

Cayce's volumes reveal another reason for us to live and live as best we can, (2) This life is an opportunity for our soul to grow and having grown in love, wisdom, and understanding to live beyond this life in the next life to come, the spiritual life. And Cayce's teachings include previous life experiences by our immortal souls and that these previous-life experiences affect our present life. As we look around the world we see advantages and disadvantages in the birth and upbringing of souls, these are a result of souls prior activities and decisions – it's karma. This new life is an opportunity for souls to resolve karma and change patterns of thought and behavior. This is true for each soul and each may also play an important role in helping other souls resolve their karma and change some of their patterns of thought and behavior.

This life is important and intentional, thus we should strive to live it as best and as long as we can.

The Scriptures state this clearly and Cayce's readings often refer to these two words in the Bible: "Choose Life." (Deuteronomy 30:19) And classical lore states, "Where there is life there is hope." This statement is often credited to Roman orator and statesman Cicero (106-43 BC). Logic suggests that if Cicero's statement is true then "Where there is hope, there should also be life." Hope is a key ingredient for a healthy, purposeful, karma-resolving incarnation.

The healthier we are, the better and the longer we can contribute to our soul growth and to the lives of others.

Here's another example from Cayce:

"Q: Please advise just how she can manifest in the earth plane to be the best channel for good?

"A: Make the body fit for the channel first! Then the spiritual may have the opportunity to manifest through. The physical must be fit, and [then] the spiritual forces may manifest the better." (295-3)

See how important physical health is. It is important for our soul's sake as well as our personality's. And it is important to other souls too. They need us more than we often know, and they need our better selves.

Sister Mary Rose McGeady (1928-2012), former president of Covenant House, the Manhattan-based home for runaway teens, also found the best reason to live: "There is no greater joy nor greater reward than to make a fundamental difference in someone's life." And Cayce supports this view: "The entity may find in the present that helping others to help themselves will bring joy, peace, happiness, contentment, and a life much worthwhile." (431-1)

If we are not physically fit then it is difficult to do good— or at least as much good as we could. We can have money, power, and fame, and yet we must have physical and mental health if we are to contribute.

—Staying Alive and Healthy—

The portion of our being that is composed of matter (i.e., flesh, blood, and bone) is so substantial and present that it is difficult to believe that *thoughts* and *attitudes* can directly affect our physical bodies. And yet our medical researchers tell us again and again that there is much evidence to prove that the state of mind, the attitude and emotions, and the expectancy of patients profoundly affects their health and healing. Oh, yes – genes play a big role for sure. Our bodies have a genetic disposition toward specific strengths and weaknesses. No one is attempting to deny that. We are simply adding the evidence that even identical twins with the same genes can have different physical conditions, and that this is due in part to their *disposition* toward life and health.

—Mind Over Matter—

"Mind-body medicine is now scientifically proven," says Herbert Benson, a cardiologist and associate professor of medicine at Harvard Medical School, who is considered a pioneer in the field. "There are literally thousands of articles on how the mind and brain affect the body." (*Alternative Medicine* by Catherine G. Davis, Twenty-First Century Books, 2012, p. 14)

And Cayce's perspective agrees, the mental state influences the physical condition. Consider this reading:

"Q: In the reading of June 3rd, it says my mental condition is paramount. Explain this in the light of how I may help my physical ailment...

"A: The explanation in this is as this: In every physical being, the whole body is made up of the atomic forces of the system, with the mind of each atom, as it is builded, supervised by the whole mental mind of the body, varied by its different phases and attributes, for, as is seen in its analyses, an atom of the body is a whole universe in itself, in the minutest state. The attitude, then, of all the attributes of the mind toward self, and the forces as manifest through same, become then paramount. As to any healing in a body, or any application of any source, nature, character, kind, or condition, is only to create that incentive IN that same atomic force to create the better condition in a body." (137-79)

As personal a part of our *being* as we feel about our bodies, they are actually *atomic structures* in which our minds and personalities function. For the most part, the atoms operate according to physical laws. It has been estimated that there are seven billion billion billion (a seven with 27 zeros after it) atoms in the human body. Roughly 65% are hydrogen, 25% oxygen, and 10% are carbon (roughly). These numerous individual atoms (protons, neutrons, and electrons) have a little consciousness of their own but they are supervised by the greater mind functioning through the brain, the master organ.

—Placebo Effect—

When a mother kisses her child's hurt, the child feels better, yet there is no medical reason for this reaction. The application of a sterile bandage creates an expectation of healing, yet there is no medical influence. When a "fake" pill is given to patients in a controlled experiment, some 32 percent of them recover, yet they received no medication. This is called the *placebo effect* or placebo response. It is believed that recovery is simply because the person has the *expectation* that it will be helpful and this expectation creates a physical, chemical response inside their bodies. Medical research has shown that "placebo effects rely on complex neurobiologic mechanisms involving neurotransmitters (e.g., endorphins, cannabinoids, and dopamine) and activation of specific, quantifiable, and relevant areas of the brain (e.g., prefrontal cortex, anterior insula, rostral anterior cingulate cortex, and amygdala in placebo analgesia). Many common medications also act through these pathways. In addition, genetic signatures of patients who are likely to respond to placebos are beginning to be identified." (*New England Journal of Medicine*: 373:8-9 July 2015)

—Expectancy—

Here's Cayce again:

"Q: Any further suggestions for the physical and spiritual improvement of this body?

"A: Keep the attitude that as the physical body is the manifestation of spiritual life and influence, it is to be used in a constructive manner as to bring hope and cheer into the lives of others. This is a reasonable service, as an appreciation, as a duty, as an opportunity for expressing the divine in self. *Be expectant* in the opportunities." (808-13, my emphasis)

And as our bodies need good food to maintain health, so do our minds and souls. According to Cayce:

"One that fills the mind, the very being, with *an expectancy* of God will see His movement, His manifestation, in the wind, the sun, the earth, the flowers, the inhabitant of the earth; and so as is builded in the body, is it to gratify just an appetite, or is it taken to fulfill ... that will the better make, the better magnify, that the body, the mind, the soul has chosen to stand for?" (341-31, my emphasis)

Along with an expectant attitude comes the power of hope.

—Hope—

We have already quoted Cicero's statement of life and hope but there is more to hope in ancient lore than we may know. For example, in mythology, Hope was the only influence that did not leave Pandora's Box and was retained when she resealed her terrible "gift" to Epimetheus. (Note:

Pandora's "box" was actually a "jar" in the original but has been misquoted over the centuries.) Here is the original:

"Only Hope was left within her unbreakable house, she remained under the lip of the jar, and did not fly away. Before [she could], Pandora replaced the lid of the jar. This was the will of aegis-bearing Zeus the Cloudgatherer."
–Hesiod's poem: *Works and Days*, (lines 96-99, ca. 700 BC)

In the 6th century BC, Theognis of Megara wrote: "Hope is the only good god remaining among mankind; the others have left and gone to Olympus."

We also have this often-quoted observation from Alexander Pope's *An Essay on Man* (1733): "Hope springs eternal in the human breast." Of course many of us would modify this statement because we've seen too much despair and depression among humanity lately. The world is severely challenged by hatred and polarization, leading to much fear and doubt about humanity's future.

But here's Cayce again, and he said this at the 8th Annual Congress of the A.R.E. in June 1939, just three months before the start of World War II—a global war that affected the entire planet: "Today, hope; today, desire. Today those things that would make you afraid are far, far away. Shadows and doubts and fears will arise in your experience, but keep before you the light of all good consciousness, of all good and perfect service to Him; and you will find that the shadows of doubt and fear will fall far behind. Let those things that cause the doubts and fears be far removed from you, through just the little kindness, the little service you may do here and there. For as you keep your mind, your body, in service that His kingdom may come in the earth, so will joy, peace, and harmony come into your experience." (262-121)

Many kindred souls have written wonderful thoughts about hope. Here are some of my favorites:

"With God all things are possible." —Jesus Christ, Matthew 19:26

"What gives me the most hope every day is God's grace; knowing that His grace is going to give me the strength for whatever I face, knowing that nothing is a surprise to God." — Rick Warren, author and pastor (1954-)

"Let your hopes, not your hurts, shape your future." — Robert H. Schuller, televangelist and writer (1926-2015)

"I always entertain great hopes." —Robert Frost, American poet (1874-1963) He also said: "In three words I can sum up everything I've learned about life: *it goes on.*"

And finally the former president of the Czech Republic, a deep thinker, caught the truth about genuine hope in this statement: "Hope is definitely not the same thing as optimism. It is not the conviction that something will turn out well, but the certainty that something makes sense regardless of how it turns out."—Vaclav Havel, writer, philosopher, and statesman (1936-2011)

In fact, this is exactly what got me into the wonderful Edgar Cayce material so long ago when I was 16 years old: *it made sense.*

—Diet and Exercise—

Of course Edgar Cayce did not ignore the needs of the physical organism. He taught:

"The physical organism is constructed in such a way and manner that if the balance is kept in the diet, in the normal activity, and the mental forces replenished, then the body should readjust itself, re-facilitate itself; making for not only resuscitation and revivifying of the necessary influences, but carrying on and reproducing itself." (1040-1)

With the proper assimilation of the nutrients needed to build and maintain our bodies and the elimination of toxins that build up in our bodies, our amazing physical vehicles will renew themselves for healthy incarnating.

Of course it is good to keep in mind that we are naturally, normally celestial, soul beings temporarily manifesting as terrestrial, physical beings – and Cayce stated this clearly:

"Spirit is the natural, the normal condition of an entity." (816-10) Spirit! Spirit is our natural, normal condition? How difficult is it to feel that truth when so profoundly associated with a flesh and bone body! It helps if we have ever known a pet well and seen it alive and well but then observed its body dead: What is no longer in our pet's body? It is that pet's spirit that we knew so well and loved. If we have seen a human alive and then dead, what has left the body? The spirit of the person that used that body has left.

Spirit is our natural, normal condition. And our spirit enters our baby body and leaves our dying body. The spirit lives on, the body is left behind.

This incarnation is an important opportunity for our spirit/soul and the spirit/souls of those with whom we share this physical life. With this in mind let's learn how to gain, regain, and maintain physical health for soulful purposes!

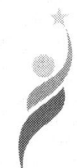

Chapter 2
The Fundamentals of
Holistic Health & Healing

When I first came across Edgar Cayce's material on health, healing, rejuvenation, and the destiny of the body (which too many of us assume to be only death), I was amazed at what I found and excited to begin using his approach in my life and the lives of my family and friends. As a boy, I had heard preachers speak of miracle healing but I had never realized how *natural* it could be until I read Cayce's material. Edgar Cayce presents a vision into what he calls, "continual life," life that continues when it is in *harmony* with the forces of Nature. When life is being lived mindfully and is lived in a balance manner, it cooperates with the universal life forces. Then the whole being hums along healthfully. When a body and mind are in cooperation and *coordination* with the natural forces in the body and the environment, then there is a rhythm that runs smoothly, bringing nourishment and rejuvenation. But when it is in contention with its various systems and subsystems, then it is at dis-ease with itself and its surroundings, and if left that way too long it leads to *disease*.

In the Cayce approach, the best way to overcome illness and disease is to preserve or restore a balanced, coordinated condition throughout the whole system.

However, if the body has developed or inherited problems, Cayce almost always approaches these with an attitude of re-creation, revitalization, revivification, and *rejuvenation.* There are no limitations, save those we put upon ourselves and upon the forces of Nature. For Cayce, the life force is that we call "spirit." Spirit is the élan vital, the Yoga *kundalini*, the "glow of life" that makes one virile and vibrant. The lack of it makes one lifeless and weak, vulnerable to all manner of illness.

The *flow* of spirit or the life forces through a body is dependent on the condition of the electrochemical *soup* of that body. It depends on the mental attitude toward health and healing. And it depends upon the openness to *spirit*, that *essence* of life throughout the infinite universe and through all of Nature. When the infinite life force is flowing through a finite, individual life, then that individual is very likely to be healthy and of sound mind, living life purposefully and contributing to the lives of others.

Cayce considered the mind to be a very important player in health and wellbeing, stating that the *thoughts* and *attitudes* of the *mind* inside that body affect the physical just as the condition of the physical affects the mind. The right thoughts, the right attitudes inside a clean, properly nourished body make for the ideal flow of the life force. This is the holism presented by Edgar Cayce. Body, mind, and spirit work together for health and healing. We cannot have wellbeing if one of these is out of sync with the others. When we seek to achieve or maintain health and rejuvenation, we need to *coordinate* the condition of our body, mind, and spirit. The three work together. Of course, if we improve one, then we positively affect the others. But we cannot have the body chemistry right while the mind's outlook is negative. And medical people will tell us that if the person does not have the spirit or will to live, then no matter what they do for the person the outcome will be negative. Body, mind, and spirit working together for the greater good of the individual is holistic health and wellness.

—A Holistic Approach—

Each of us is a spirit with a mind incarnate in a physical body. Therefore, awareness of the mental and spiritual forces is as important as attention to physical foods, exercises, medicines, and therapies.

Here's one of Cayce's statements on this:

"Bringing normalcy and a revivifying of purposes, desires or ambitions – the body WHOLE must be taken into consideration; that is, the physical, the mental and the spiritual attributes of the body." (1189-2; Note: His stenographer explained that when his voice rose in volume, she then recorded the word in all-capital letters to give the word emphasis—as in the sentence where the word WHOLE is in capital letters because he raised his voice when he said it.)

Here are two more Cayce statements:

"These bespeak of something innate within self that bespeaks of the abilities of the soul, mind, and body to revivify and rejuvenate itself as to an ideal." (578-2)

Holding an ideal purpose for regaining health and living life is key to moving the body toward that goal. More on setting and living by an ideal will be explained on page 32.

Here's another Cayce insight:

"To be sure, as it has been indicated again and again, there is that within the physical forces of the body which may be revivified or rejuvenated, if it is kept in a constructive way and manner. This requires, necessarily, the proper thinking, the proper living, the proper application of those influences in the experience of an entity in its associations with everything about a body." (681-2)

His approach is clearly body-mind-spirit, thus holistic by its very definition.

—Cayce's Causes for Illness—

Here are Cayce's primary causes for illness:

- A diet lacking the nutrients needed to maintain a healthy body;

- Poor assimilation of the nutrients needed by the body;
- Poor eliminations of the toxins that build up inside a body;
- Improper acid-alkaline balance in the body (mostly due to too much acidity);
- Incoordination of the nervous systems of the body (the cerebrospinal or central nervous system and the autonomic nervous system which is composed of the sympathetic and the parasympathetic systems – more on these later);
- Imbalance in the circulatory system of the body. The circulatory system or *cardiovascular* system is an organic system that permits blood to circulate so it may transport nutrients, oxygen, carbon dioxide, hormones, and blood cells to and from the cells throughout the body to provide nourishment, fight diseases, stabilize temperature and pH (the acid/alkaline balance), and maintain a stable and relatively constant condition of health. The circulatory system is comprise of two separate systems: the cardiovascular system that distributes blood and the lymphatic system that distributes lymph, a fluid containing infection-fighting white blood cells throughout the body;
- Malfunction of the glandular system of the body, especially the endocrine glands that generate the powerful hormones that send messages directly through the blood stream to various cells and organs for ideal functioning and/or adjusting to changes in the environment;
- Of course he includes *infection*: this is the invasion and multiplication of harmful agents such as bacteria, viruses, and parasites that are not normally present in the body;
- Overexertion from too little rest, inadequate sleep, insufficient recreation, and not enough renewal time (both physically *and* mentally).

To this list Cayce adds these usually not considered causes:
- Despair and heartache to such a degree that the person's entire system is affected negatively;

- Too much anger, hatred, and other dark attitudes and emotions;
- Karma – yes, Cayce considers that the soul may be carrying a negative influence that occurred early in this incarnation or even prior to this incarnation. Even Jesus was asked by his disciples why a man was *born* blind: "Did he or his parents do something to cause this?" Now since the man was *born* blind that would indicate that the cause occurred *prior* to this incarnation. (John 9:2)

As you can see from this list Cayce covers a wide range of causes for illness and disease, many we already know about and consider but some that we do not normally regard. And in most of these causes there is clearly a preventative way to avoid the problems or recover from them.

Let's take a brief look at our body, mind, spirit arrangement.

—The Body—

For true healing and health to occur one must take into consideration all *subsystems* of the total body. Within a body, Cayce strives for *overall* improvement in a balanced and coordinated manner, never focusing on just one portion of the system but seeing the system as just that, *an integrated system!* The body is an *organism* that functions as a singular whole. It's parts (atoms, cells, tissue, organs, etc.) are woven into the fabric of the whole—not independent of the whole. Now we are speaking of the *ideal* healthy state. One can function reasonably well missing a part or having a malfunctioning part, but even in these cases the contribution of that part must be accounted for by supplements or other parts that assume the role played in the overall functioning of the organism.

—The Mind—

Beyond the body Cayce insist that true healing and wellness must include the condition and activity of the mind. Especially when attempting to improve the body. During eating, exercising, receiving treatment, and taking supplements or medications one must be positive, *expectant,* and mindful of why they are doing what they are doing and how it is going to contribute to their health and wellbeing.

"Keep the mental and the spiritual forces active during the applications; not done as rote! Know within self something is being accomplished through the applications." (1158-1)

The key word in this last Cayce statement is "within." The coordination of body-mind-spirit begins *within* us. As most doctors confess, the ultimate decision for health is *within* their patient. One can apply all the miracles of modern science, psychology, or mystical religion but unless something inside that person is stirred to live, to rejuvenate, little may be accomplished.

—Spiritual Forces—

As much as God has been bashed my humanity's religious dogma, prejudice, segregation, hatred of others, wars to kill others, and so on, the *spiritual forces* must be a part of our approach to healing and health. This is not so much religious as it is spiritual. One does not have to believe in God but one has to believe in spiritual forces or the *life essence* seen throughout the universe. Often called the élan vital, kundalini, ch'i, and life energy, Edgar Cayce referred to them as the spiritual forces, teaching that they *are* the healing forces. He never backs off of this principle. Here's one of his comments:

"In the present there may be gained within self the raising within self that consciousness of the at-onement with the spiritual forces that may revivify, regenerate, arouse that of health and happiness even under the adverse conditions in materiality." (618-3)

Bringing ourselves into "at-onement" with the life forces, the spiritual forces, is required. Think of our body as a musical instrument. In the case of illness it is out of tune. When it is healthy it is in tune. Consider the universal life force as an orchestra, and we are an individual instrument in that orchestra. When we tune ourselves with the universal essence of life, then we are in harmony, causing the symphony without *and within* to sound ideal.

An orchestra tunes itself to a very particular frequency, usually 440 hertz, a note known as A 440. The note is played by the oboist, and the rest of the orchestra tunes their instruments to match it. The oboe leads the tuning because of all the instruments in the orchestra it is least affected by humidity or other weather conditions. Cayce indicates that the *spiritual essence* of our being is least affected by the chemical soup and electrical vibrations of our human body and our circumstances. Therefore, to get into harmony and perfect pitch, we need to feel the frequency of the infinite spirit of life! Then we must tune our instrument (our body) to that frequency.

In this instruction we just read Cayce declares that this will work "even under the adverse conditions in materiality!" Thus, nothing physical can stand in the way of revivification, regeneration, and arousal of our health and happiness – except ourselves. This is not to say that under all circumstances this will be easy. Life is often difficult. Surroundings are often not ideal. But if we truly strive to tune our instrument to the life force within us, then little by little, day by day, we will get on the right pitch, the right frequency.

Cayce adds that these forces are *natural* not supernatural as some would teach. And they are open to all souls, no matter what culture, race, nationality, or belief system they hold, or even if they have no belief system. The infinite life force flows to any who open themselves to it and attempt to tune themselves to its life-giving, life-sustaining vibration. There is one requirement: *quietness*.

"The revivifying forces ... are the NATURAL sources of energies through quietness within any given activity that makes for strengthening for resistances of every nature in a physical body." (587-5)

Of course Cayce encouraged the enlistment of the Creator of Life, the Source of Life, which we call God. However, his view of God was much bigger than that of most religions and people. He saw a Universal Consciousness and Life Force that collectively sustains all beings, all emanations of life – minerals, vegetables, animals, and humans (even discarnate beings, such as angels, fairies, the elementals). The only religious principle he held to was *one* Universal Consciousness (one God) and that all emanations from this original One were *family!* Everyone, everything belonged to one family, despite the many attempts to teach otherwise. He encouraged us to see others as we see ourselves, to love others as we love ourselves. On the surface there are differences. And there are different motivations and moral standards, but within the core of everything and everyone is a central essence that is from the same Source of Life.

With this in mind, we will now look at his teachings to include God in our health restoration and maintenance.

Consider this teaching of his:

"The revivifying influences will give your inner self that which will create, that which will build in the body, as you hold to that you know within your self – that He, the Giver of all good and perfect gifts, is renewing your strength and your life within you; and that you will USE same in His service so long as the days are given unto you for your activities in this material world. And we will find STRENGTH being built in your body as the stamina of steel! And, as the vital forces renew your vitality in your body, USE your mental self." (716-2)

From Cayce's perspective God's service is to help bring about harmony, cooperation, and coordination throughout the whole of the creation. The spirit of love and caring is the right vibration and the right attitude for bringing ourselves into God's service. Thus the two great commandments of love God (the Life Force, Source of Life, and Creative Forces) and love one another (the emanations from the One Source) are key to our being in "His service," as Cayce stated in that reading.

For Cayce, God is not so much a personal being as an infinite, eternal Spirit from which all beings have emanated and in which they have their existence. We may often feel alone, disconnected, and left to ourselves, but if we can grasp even a tiny sense of our unbreakable connection to the Life Force of the infinite, eternal Spirit, then our healing begins! I am not saying that we will not have to do some specific physical and mental work to improve, we will, but with this connected awareness to the Source of life, our efforts will have better results.

—Healing and Health Comes from Within—

This is perhaps the most difficult concept for us to grasp. Despite the applications of medicines, hi-tech machines, foods, and physical manipulations, the body actually receives its ultimate healing and wellness *from the forces within it*. All these other elements are simply catalyst or stimulants to encourage the bodily forces to bring about a healthy condition.

"From whence comes the healing?" Cayce asks, "Whether there is administered a drug, a correcting or an adjustment of a subluxation, or the alleviating of a strain upon the muscles, or the revivifying through electrical forces; they are ONE, and the healing comes from WITHIN! Not by the method does the healing come, though the consciousness of the individual IS such that this or that method IS the one that is more effective in the individual case in arousing the forces from within. But the METHODS are NOT ideals. The IDEAL must be kept in the proper SOURCE." (969-1)

Here Cayce is commenting on the truth that the *method* is not the miracle. Yet, he acknowledges that the method is critical because of the *belief system*, the mind-set of the individual, and that must be considered when deciding what method to use. As Cayce once explained, a quinine consciousness cannot be healed of malaria with anything but quinine – for that person has set the condition for healing and recovery *in their mind!* (5211-1) Nevertheless, it is not the quinine that is the healer, but the mind within the person that believes quinine is the healing substance for them. The source of healing is *within* us.

Now this is not to say that a very persuasive person, such as a doctor with a good reputation and powerful skills of persuasion, could not change a patient's mind, and thereby break through their mindset. Or that loved ones cannot affect healing just by their trusted presence. It can. I have seen it change an ill person almost immediately upon the entry of the loved and trusted presence.

If we realize this, and become *mindful,* meaning *consciously aware* of our inner thoughts, beliefs, and attitudes, then we can make *significant* changes in our overall condition. In many cases *we know what we need* in order to recover!

—The Right Ideal and Purpose—

If we came to Cayce for guidance, he would not immediately tell us to pray, meditate, or seek a dream; he'd *first* tell us to *set an ideal,* a *standard* by which we could measure the *value* of whatever we do or intend to do. The ideal is like a pole star by which we guide our lives and decisions. Rather than letting the circumstances of life rule us, we set the direction, the purpose and the ultimate condition sought; then everything moves toward realizing that Ideal. Even when circumstances are hard against us, we, like the captain of a great sailing ship, tack against that wind, ever moving toward our ideal, even if we have to do it in a zig-zag manner (tacking against the wind) – and when the wind eases or changes direction, we'll be in a better position than if we had simply let the circumstances (the wind currents) of our life take us wherever *they* would.

This is the power of an ideal. It helps us understand why we do something, what we desire to realize or become, and gives us a measuring rod by which to judge the elements of a decision or activity that better lead to the ideal.

Cayce: "Begin to PLAN as to what the body will DO when and AS the improvements come. Not only be good, be good FOR SOMETHING! Hold to that which is Truth!" (572-5)

Here's how Cayce says our minds use our ideals, and somewhat surprisingly, he says our desires often knock our ideals off track:

"The mind uses its spiritual ideals to build upon. And the mind also uses the material desires as the destructive channels, or it is the interference by the material desires that prevents a body and a mind from keeping in perfect accord with its ideal.

"Thus, these continue ever in the material plane to be as warriors one with another. Physical emergencies or physical conditions may oft be used as excuses, or as justifications for the body choosing to do this or that. Ought these things so to be, according to your ideal?

"Then, the more important, the most important experience of this or any individual entity is to first know what *is* the ideal – spiritually.

"Who and what is thy pattern?

"Throughout the experience of man in the material world, at various seasons and periods, teachers or 'would-be' teachers have come; setting up certain forms or certain theories as to manners in which an individual shall control the appetites of the body or of the mind, so as to attain to some particular phase of development.

"There has also come a Teacher who was bold enough to declare Himself as the Son of the living God. He set no rules of appetite. He set no rules of ethics, other than, 'As you would that men should do to you, do you even so to them,' and to know 'Inasmuch as you do it unto the least of these, your brethren, you do it unto your Maker." He declared that the kingdom of heaven is within each individual entity's consciousness." (357-13)

And again:

"First, know what is your own ideal. Not as to what others may do for you, but what is the ideal way of individuals to live among themselves? What do you believe as to those things pertaining to the relationship of self, as an individual, to the Creative Forces or God? What manner of expression should self give as in its relationships to same? In whom have you believed? What is the source of your faith, of your hope? And then, so live, so act among others, that you are a living example of that you believe." (1755-3)

Cayce was asked for help with this:

"Q-5. Will you give further enlightenment to help accomplish this desire?

"A-5. The basis of every entity's activity should be the placing of an ideal in the experiences of self. Not an idol, not an idea, not a position even that may be attained in the earth's experience by earthly activities; for to attain that which is wholly desired in the mental abilities of an entity is to become stale and self-centered. Then, naturally, the retrogression would ensue.

"Hence, the attaining of that which makes for the better and greater development in the earth's experience is to be wholly dependent, in the mental-spiritual activities, upon the will of the Creator, or Creative Forces, that may manifest through every activity of self; making self then a channel day by day in the direction that is set as the ideal of the *soul*, not of the mental mind.

"Each activity is a manifestation of the forces that emanate from the universal, or the consciousness of the living God! Individuals' activity upon that, by their construction of same, makes it hell or heaven!

"Then, each soul should see more and more constructively in regard to the most destructive influences in an activity! One that does not accomplish this loses, or besets self to self's own undoing!" (270-31)

And again he warns:

"Do not let, or allow, disappointments to persuade or misdirect the intent and purpose as it is innately manifested in your experience." (1968-2)

Of course, for Cayce the ideal would be in the spiritual forces, for they are the source of health and healing.

"Life is the manifestation of that Divine which is worshiped as God. Hence each soul-entity is a portion of same, with that privilege through the experiences in materiality to manifest an ideal and thus grow in grace, in knowledge, in faith, in hope, in love; that the entity, the soul, may be one with the Creative Forces – that should be the ideal of every soul." (1082-3)

And again:

"Put your ideal in those things that bespeak of the continuity of life; the regeneration of the spiritual body, the revivifying of the temporal body for SPIRITUAL purposes, that the seed may go forth even as the Teacher gave, "Sin no more, but present your body as a living sacrifice; holy, acceptable unto Him, for it is a reasonable service." (969-1)

—The Right Mental Attitude—

Two people can do exactly the same things toward rejuvenation and wellness, and get different results. So often the influencing force in these cases is their attitude. One is hopeful and expectant, the other doubts or feels unworthy. Attitude is a powerful, unseen influence in the outcome of any activity.

"To be sure, there should be rather that expectant attitude of the body ... for unless there is the expectancy, unless there is hope, the mind's outlook becomes a drag, a drug on one that is being attacked from within by the dis-eases of a physical body." (572-5)

"DO NOT become morose. Do not doubt the abilities of those influences in the spiritual life to meet the needs of the body physically, mentally, spiritually, and we will revivify these things." (458-2)

"Nothing save self stands in the way of the entity MAKING or becoming a channel of blessings to many! For the entity may be assured, for the entity will find, nothing in heaven or hell or earth may separate you from the knowledge and the use of the I AM PRESENCE within, save selfishness – or self!" (440-20)

"Hence mind over matter is not to be lightly spoken of, nor is there any disparaging remark to be made as to the ability of the body-physical to be revivified, resuscitated, spiritualized such that there is no reaction that may not be revivified." (1152-5)

"For HE hath shown the way – not by some mysterious fluid, not by some unusual vibration, but by the simple method of LIVING that which is LIFE itself. THINK no evil; HEAR no evil. And as the Truth flows as a stream of life through the Mind in all its phases or aspects, and purifies same, so will it purify and revivify and rejuvenate the body. For once this effacement urge is overcome, then may there begin the rejuvenation." (294-183)

Notice "this effacement urge" and how it fits with what our society has been learning about poor self-esteem. Critical experiences form our beliefs about ourselves, and usually occur early in life. What we saw, heard and experienced in childhood, in our family, in the community, and at school have a profound influence on the way we see ourselves. Sometimes negative beliefs about ourselves are caused by experiences later in life, such as workplace intimidation, abusive relationships, persistent stress or hardship, or traumatic life events. Becoming mindful of any such impact on our self-esteem is important to healing the vibrations of our body and removing negativity and stress in our minds and thoughts.

"Mind IS the master, yet physical conditions need the activity of those impulses through same that may regenerate or revivify the abilities for reproduction of self through the afflicted or disturbed areas of the body." (2529-1)

"It may appear long, but – keep that attitude of being the channel through which more love of the divine nature may be given, even as ye would be SHOWN that towards the ways and manners for the helpfulness in the material physical body." (1199-3)

"The destruction of the blood forces [is] by SUPPRESSION of self in a mental manner. Hence, the necessity of directing and interesting self in a FAD, or even a FANCY, and keeping self interested in same, as well as correcting the physical conditions." (5554-2)

See how the physical corrections need to be made but the mind and its interests in living must also be involved in and excited about living!

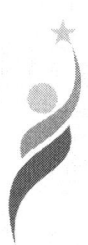

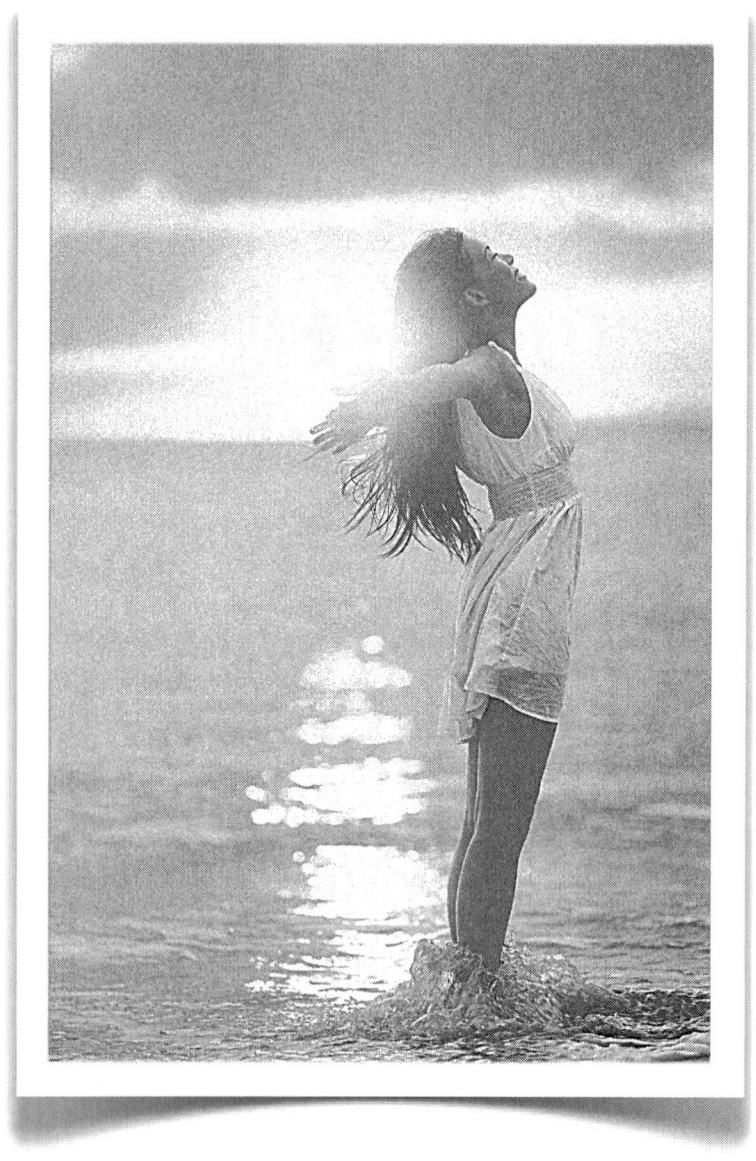

Rejuvenation!

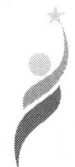

Chapter 3
REJUVENATION
Rebuilding Our Bodies

—The Body can Reproduce Itself—

Among the many amazing concepts in the volumes of Cayce's channeled material are discourses on the human body's wonderful restorative powers. In this chapter we review some of these teachings.

"Q: Is it possible for our bodies to be rejuvenated in this incarnation?

"A: Possible. The body is an atomic structure, the units of energy around which there are the movements of atomic forces that are ever the pattern of a universe. Then, when these atoms are made to conform or rely upon or to be one with the spiritual import, the spiritual activity, then they revivify, then they make for constructive forces." (262-85)

"The physical organism is constructed in such a way and manner that if the balance is kept in the diet, in the normal activity, and the mental forces replenished, then the body should readjust itself, re-facilitate itself; making for not only resuscitation and revivifying of the necessary influences but carrying on and reproducing itself." (1040-1)

"The body should in its elements be able, as it does continually, to reproduce itself; making for not only revivifying or resuscitating forces but keeping nominally alive." (1038-1)

"If there will be gained that consciousness, there need not be ever the necessity of a physical organism aging ... seeing this, feeling this, knowing this, ye will find that not only does the body become revivified, but by creating in every atom of its being the knowledge of the activity of this Creative Force ... spirit, mind, body are renewed." (1299-1)

"How is the way shown by the Master? What is the promise in Him? The last to be overcome is death. Death of what? The soul cannot die, for it is of God. The body may be revivified, rejuvenated – and it is to that end it may, the body, TRANSCEND the earth and its influences." (262-85)

If we accept the principles in these statements, then health and a long life are a matter of applying these principles in our bodies, minds and spirits. For Cayce, all three of these aspects of our being have to be in cooperation and full activity with one another before true healing and rejuvenation can take hold.

—The Seven-Year Cycle of Renewal—

According to the Cayce readings, the body rebuilds itself in its entirety every seven years. Therefore, no matter what problem we have, if we would apply ourselves to changing it, and work patiently throughout the seven-year cycle, our bodies would have rebuilt every cell according to this new ideal, this new goal, this new hope.

"Every seven years there is performed an entire renewal of the whole structural or anatomical body." (887-4)

"In this particular body ... the system will produce that which will enable the body to continue without any let-down for a period of another cycle to three cycles. Then, before there is any real let-down in the abilities of the body, there should be at least twenty-one more years of activity." [7 years per cycle, times 3 cycles, equals 21 years] (1064-1, an adult, but age at time of reading was unknown)

Research has found this 7-year cycle to be *mostly* true. Investigation into the renewal cycle began in the 1950s; long after Cayce had passed on in 1945. The research took on even more intensity around the year 2000, and in 2005 Nicolas Wade published his attention-getting article in the New York Times, "Your Body is Younger than You Think" (August 2, 2005). In this article he presented much of what has been discovered concerning the body's process of sloughing off old cells and generating new, fresh cells. Wade also showed how our DNA stays the same as it was when we were born but constant dividing to make new cells explains how aging occurs. In other words, aging is not a cellular problem per se, it is a DNA issue. And on July 14, 2007 National Public Radio (NPR) presented the show, "Atomic Tune-Up: How the Body Rejuvenates Itself." On June 24, 2013 *Science Update* published "Bombs and Brain Cells," in which we learned that a small population of our brain cells remain *permanently* young, renewing themselves continually. The research team estimated that we generate around 1400 new neurons *every day*. However, for some unknown reason yet to be discovered the newborn brain cells do not appear to live long and there are more dying than being born – thus aging occurs.

—The Genetics of Aging—
Take a Brief University Course with Me

Research has discovered that a major cause of aging is what they call "oxidative stress," meaning DNA, proteins, and lipids are damaged over time by oxidants. Oxidants result from metabolism, which is the chemical processes by which cells produce the substances and energy needed to sustain life. Oxidants generate "free radicals," which are atoms or groups of atoms with an odd (unpaired) number of electrons. Free radicals are the unstable molecules that react with other substances in our bodies that damage cells or create abnormal ones, such as cancer cells. Free radicals are unavoidable and are created naturally so our body can perform its everyday functions. They are necessary for some processes.

Fortunately our bodies naturally produce another category of compounds called *antioxidants*. This is why we hear so much about supplements that are antioxidants, such as vitamins A, C, and E and the minerals calcium, zinc, magnesium, and selenium.

In a healthy body oxidants and antioxidants maintain a balance. If this ratio shifts towards pro-oxidants then we have oxidative stress. This oxidative stress may be either mild or severe depending on the extent of shift. It remains the cause of disease and aging. Much research is being done on this topic and as more reports are publicized we may come to have a clearer understanding of how to keep our bodies healthier longer.

An interesting discovery has already added much to our understanding. Inside the nucleus of a cell our genes are arranged along an entwined double-strand of molecules of DNA called *chromosomes*. At the ends of the chromosomes are stretches of DNA called *telomeres*, which *protect* our genetic information while making it possible for our cells to divide and produce new cells.

Telomeres maybe compared to the plastic tips on shoelaces because they keep the ends of our chromosomes from fraying or sticking to each other. Surprisingly, each time a cell divides the telomeres get shorter. When they get too short, then the cell can no longer divide. This shortening process is associated with aging, cancer, and a higher risk of death. So telomeres also have been compared with a bomb fuse ("Bombs and Brain Cells" *Science Update*).

For example, in white blood cells telomeres are about 8,000 base pairs in newborn bodies to 3,000 base pairs in adult bodies and then as low as 1,500 in elderly bodies. During cell division an average cell loses 30 to 200 base pairs from the ends of its telomeres.

Cells normally can divide only about 50 to 70 times. While telomere shortening has been linked to the aging process,

Geneticist Richard Cawthon and colleagues at the University of Utah and others cannot yet determine whether shorter telomeres are just a sign of aging – like gray hair – or actually *contribute* to aging.

Scientists have been able to use *telomerase* in the lab to keep human cells dividing far beyond their normal limit, and the cells do not become cancerous. If we use enzymes that add nucleotides to telomeres to "immortalize" human cells, then we may be able to mass produce cells for transplantation, including insulin-producing cells to cure diabetes, muscle cells for treating muscular dystrophy, cartilage cells for certain kinds of arthritis, and skin cells for healing severe burns and wounds. An unlimited supply of normal human cells grown in the laboratory would also help efforts to test new drugs and gene therapies.

Human lifespan has increased since the 1600s, when the average lifespan was 30 years. By 2012 the average U.S. life expectancy was nearly 79. Reasons for the increase include sewers and other sanitation measures, antibiotics, clean water, refrigeration, vaccines, and other medical efforts to prevent children and babies from dying, improve diets, and provide better health care.

Some scientists predict that the average life expectancy will continue to increase, although many doubt the average will ever be much higher than 90. But a few say vastly longer lifespans are possible. Geneticist Richard Cawthon says that if all processes of aging could be eliminated and oxidative stress damage repaired, "one estimate is people could live 1,000 years." Now that takes us back to Old Testament ages: Adam lived to be 930, Methuselah 969, and Noah 950!

—Oxidative Stress—

Leonard Smith, M.D., a gastrointestinal, vascular surgeon developed the following guide:

"There are many different processes and substances that damage cells and contribute to oxidative stress including:

•Toxic chemical compounds and pollutants in your body

•Hydrogenated fats

•All kinds of pollution, including air, water, and food

•Oils that have been heated to very high temperatures [as in deep-fried foods]

•Cigarette smoke, directly inhaled or secondhand

•Dehydration

•Too much sugar

•Too much animal protein in your diet

•Geophysical stress like living near power lines or waste dumps

•Microbial imbalance, including bacterial, fungal and viral infections

•Preservatives in your food

•Drugs (over the counter and prescription)

•Artificial food colorings and flavorings

•Plastics and phthalates

•Chemical cleaning supplies

•Chlorinated water that you drink, shower in or swim in

•Alcohol

•Pesticides in your food

•Radiation exposure

•Psychological and emotional stress

Your body generates free radicals every day, but you don't have to let free radical damage cause premature aging and disease!" (Source: BodyEcology.com)

—Understanding Inflammation—

Chronic Inflammation

Our amazing bodies naturally become inflamed in response to injury or infection, revealing this in the form of swelling, heat, redness, and pain. The process includes increased blood flow with an influx of white blood cells and other chemical substances that facilitate healing. This is the body's way of getting more immune activity into an area that needs to fend off infection or heal from injury. And it is an important and natural function of our bodies.

However, there is another kind of inflammation that is not healthy and is a cause of aging and disease. It is called *chronic inflammation*. It is often imperceptible because it is a low-level inflammation that wears on our body over time. Now one's genetics plays a part in one's body being inclined to chronic inflammation but so does a sedentary lifestyle (little to no exercise), too much stress and toxins. The food we eat also has a huge impact on our body's state of inflammation. Some medical researchers believe that the single most important thing we can do to counter chronic inflammation is to stop eating refined, processed, and manufactured foods – eat real foods, as fresh as possible and with the least amount of processing. And guess which foods are anti-inflammatory – *fruits and vegetables!*

—Detoxing Our Bodies the Cayce Way—

A new baby's cells are filled with vitality and little to no toxins. In a baby's body life is flowing with a sparkle. If the child is nursing on mother's milk then even its poops don't smell! How clean is that? Wouldn't it be nice to at least have some of our own baby-body purity back? Edgar Cayce says we can get close to that!

Our bodies are amazing but they do need some help from time to time. Two features of a healthy body are proper *assimilation* of the nutrients needed to feed its cells and the *elimination* of toxins that build up in the body. This is especially true if the body is not being active, because in that case fluids and toxins pool in the body and do not get to our elimination systems.

—Our Elimination Systems—

We have 4 systems devoted to elimination of toxins and dross. They are:
- Skin & Sweat Glands
- Lungs & Breath

•Digestive System & Bowel Movements

•Urinary System & Urine

As we can quickly see if we are not properly functioning in any one of these systems then toxins and dross back up in our body and we begin to decline in health and freshness.

Eliminations in the Edgar Cayce teachings were very important to health!

6 Quick Tips for Improving Eliminations

1. Chew our food! Sounds natural but it is not. Cayce was clear about how chewing food prepares it for easier digestion. For example, saliva contains the enzyme *amylase* that breaks some starches down into maltose and dextrin. Thus, digestion of food begins in the mouth, even before it reaches the stomach. Saliva and chewing also creates the "bolus," a soft mass of chewed food that makes digestion easier and more complete. Here is one example from Cayce's files: ""For each and every body there should be the thorough mastication [chewing]. For if this is done the activity of the glands in the mouth and the salivary glands is such as to keep the throat and the bronchi in a much healthier condition. Bolting food or swallowing it by the use of liquids produces more colds than ANY ONE activity of a diet! Even milk or water should be CHEWED two to three times before taken into the stomach itself, for this makes for the proper assimilation of the lacteal activity in the system; and when being acted upon by the gastric flow of the hydrochlorics in the duodenum area, it is better assimilated and gives more value in the whole of the body." (808-3) Note: Hydrochloric acid is found naturally in human gastric acid.

2. Do not mix so much fluid with the food by drinking while eating. This allows the powerful digestive fluids to be at their full strength when processing ingested food.

3. Eat Real Food. I know this sounds surprising but too much of our ingested meals are processed. Processed foods often contain what is known as "empty" calories. Calories are a

way of describing how much energy our bodies get from eating a food. The term empty calories applies to food such as solid fats and those with added sugars that provide little or no nutrition. Many of us eat far too many processed foods that provide little real energy. It is better to eat foods that Nature created and as fresh as possible.

4. Eat liver-healthy foods because the liver removes harmful material from the bloodstream and plays an important role in proper digestion. The liver-loving foods are leafy green vegetables like leafy lettuce and spinach, cruciferous veggies like broccoli and Brussels sprouts, and avocados, lemons, grapefruit, walnuts, garlic, and even green tea. Purifying the blood system is an important step. Here's Cayce:

"The body rebuilds itself CONSTANTLY, through what? The BLOOD supply!" (683-3)

"In the blood supply of this body – as in most bodies – lies the life and extenuation of life, the abilities to create and to eliminate from the system destructive forces, as well as within same create constructive, resuscitating, revivifying forces within the body." (443-2)

"Gradually, as the strength and resistance and the bloodstream becomes renewed and revivified, the eliminations and the drosses become less and less a portion of the problem." (1173-1)

5. Hydrate! We hear it all the time but how many of us actually drink 6 to 8 glasses of water a day as Edgar Cayce recommended (that's 48 to 64 ounces). And he wanted us to "chew" the water so as to mix our saliva with it before we swallow.

6. Reduce stress, inactivity, and emotionally disturbing TV, movies, thoughts, and situations. We each have a free-will and can make better choices for our health. Nothing truly stands in our way but ourselves. Of course habits and patterns of behavior are difficult to change. Whatever it takes we can

with patience and persistence overcome or change our daily experiences for the better.

Cayce wanted a balanced life, meaning going out into life and the lives of others while also budgeting time to go within to tune to the renewing forces of the Spirit within us. He wanted recreation with rest, study with reflection, selflessness with self-discovery, knowledge with application. Using these we should find ourselves healthier and happier – even a bit younger!

What is important for our purposes here is that our bodies know how to renew themselves. If we hold a mindful awareness of this process and can maintain a balanced ratio in our bodies between oxidants and antioxidants, then we can improve every 7 years and thereby build and maintain a healthier body.

There will be some specific therapies for improving the functioning of our elimination systems later in this book.

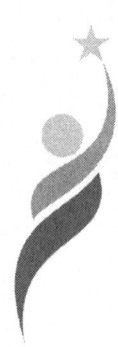

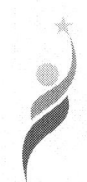

Chapter 4
The Mechanics of
Health, Healing, and Rejuvenation

Since our souls live in and express through these physical bodies it is a good idea to get to know these bodies and how they best function. Cayce conveyed volumes on how the body operates best. Let's look at some of his teachings on this important subject.

—Balance and Coordination are Required—

"To be rejuvenated, the body must be kept in a condition of construction; to ever find that the heart, the digestive organs' combination of elimination and assimilation, the hair, the scalp, the nasal, the eye, the ear, the throat, the bronchi, the lungs, the structural forces of the body work as a UNIT, or as ONE! And then we may find, and do find, the body BUILDING, ever." (681-2)

"There must be kept a body-balance." (681-2)

"There is more than one manner of eliminating the conditions, but inasmuch as there needs to be the reviving, the revivifying and the coordination of the vibratory forces through the body – we find these as we will give would be the more preferable ways and manners for making for the corrections to be of a permanent nature; thus revivifying the whole of the body." (1196-1)

"There may be created that balance of cooperation and coordination throughout the physical forces of the body, revivifying those disturbances to a constructive activity, rather than a tearing down; and creating those balances in the coordination of the mental with the spiritual for the material activity." (1173-8)

"As there is the revivifying of the whole system, this [ailment] should take on a different condition, as the GENERAL condition is helped, see?" (366-3)

—Ionizing and Re-Ionizing—

Before we go any further we need some understanding a little about electrolytes, which are ions, and the process of electrolysis. We don't need a deep college-level course but jsut enough to comprehend Cayce's teaching. Besides, electrolytes are very important to our health. So let's begin with a section from Philip Schatz *Anatomy and Physiology* textbook:

"The body contains a large variety of ions, or electrolytes, which perform a variety of functions. Some ions assist in the transmission of electrical impulses along cell membranes in neurons and muscles. Other ions help to stabilize protein structures in enzymes. Still others aid in releasing hormones from endocrine glands. All of the ions in plasma contribute to the osmotic balance that controls the movement of water between cells and their environment. Electrolytes in living systems include sodium, potassium, chloride, bicarbonate, calcium, phosphate, magnesium, copper, zinc, iron, manganese, molybdenum, copper, and chromium. In terms of body functioning, six electrolytes are most important: sodium, potassium, chloride, bicarbonate, calcium, and phosphate. These six ions aid in nerve excitability, endocrine secretion, membrane permeability, buffering body fluids, and controlling the movement of fluids between compartments. These ions enter the body through the digestive tract. More than 90 percent of the calcium and phosphate that enters the body is incorporated into bones and teeth, with bone serving as a mineral reserve for these ions. In the event that calcium and phosphate are needed for other functions, bone tissue can be broken down to supply the blood and other tissues with these minerals. Phosphate is a normal constituent of nucleic acids; hence, blood levels of phosphate will increase whenever nucleic acids are broken down. Excretion of ions occurs mainly through the kidneys, with lesser amounts lost in sweat and in feces. Excessive sweating may cause a significant loss, especially of sodium and chloride. Severe vomiting or diarrhea will cause a loss of chloride and bicarbonate ions. Adjustments in respiratory and renal [kidney] functions allow the body to regulate the levels of these ions in the ECF." ECF is an abbreviation for *extracellular fluid*. (Source: philxschatz.com/anatomy-book/contents/m46414.html)

Okay, that wasn't so bad was it? Basically, electrolytes are minerals in our bodies that have an electric charge. They are in our blood, urine, and bodily fluids. Maintaining the right balance of electrolytes is important to our blood chemistry, muscle action, and bodily processes. Sodium, calcium, potassium, chlorine, phosphate and magnesium are all electrolytes. And these are found in our foods and liquids. Levels of electrolytes in our bodies can become too low or too high. That can happen when the amount of water in our bodies changes, causing dehydration or over-hydration. Dramatic changes may occur as a result of medicines, vomiting, diarrhea, sweating or kidney problems. Problems most often occur with levels of sodium, potassium, or calcium.

Those of us who have had children know how quickly their little bodies can become ion depleted – we go to the store and buy a bottle of liquid with electrolytes to replace the electrolytes lost through dehydration, vomiting, or diarrhea. Unfortunately, modern products are often contaminated with ingredients that harm more then help, such as dextrose, salt, artificial flavors, artificial sweeteners and food color dyes. Buyers beware for most ALL of the popular brands for electrolytes sold in our grocery stores are filled with these! (Even the National Football League uses a brand derived from petrochemicals and using color dyes. These dyes have been found to inhibit mitochondrial respiration, which is the powerhouse in our cells to convert nutrients to energy! Fortunately, there are products made with some wisdom and their electrolytes come from calcium, magnesium, and bicarbonate, with vitamin B6 – important in the absorption of magnesium. These nutrients and electrolytes are often added to purified water, carbonated water, or mineral water. For more on this go to:

paleoedge.com/best-and-worst-electrolyte-drinks/

As we read on we are going to find Cayce focusing on ionizing the blood and even the nerve forces in our bodies. Hopefully, we now have a better understanding of what he is seeking and how he gets the ionization from our foods, beverages, and other means, such as fresh air.

However, we begin with the importance of our blood chemistry and how it is the main source of renewal and extension of life!

—The Blood—

Here we repeat his insight into how important the condition of our blood supply is:

"The body rebuilds itself CONSTANTLY, through what? The BLOOD supply!" (683-3)

"In the blood supply of this body (as in most bodies…) lies the life and extenuation of life, the abilities to create and to eliminate from the system destructive forces, as well as within same create constructive, resuscitating, revivifying forces within the body." (443-2)

"Gradually, as the strength and resistance and the bloodstream becomes renewed and revivified, the eliminations and the drosses become less and less a portion of the problem." (1173-1)

—Re-Ionizing the Blood—

"Q: Have I sufficient magnetism?

"A: This rises and falls easily, owing to the lack of ionization through the system. Hence the low electrical and vibratory form of activity necessary in the body." (1811-1)

"This re-ionizing of the bloodstream, the revivifying of the flows to the internal as well as the external circulation, should revitalize these [weaknesses of the body]." (1299-1)

"The use of the Radio-Active Appliance would RE-IONIZE the system, if this is used of evenings before retiring. Not AFTER retiring, but BEFORE retiring; while the body meditates use the Appliance." (189-4)

More information on the Radio-Active Appliance is coming in the Therapies chapter but for now know that it has nothing to do with nuclear energy. It is more like a radio wave device than nuclear fission!

"There must be kept a body-balance, then. Hence, ionizing of the energies from all the radial forces about the superficial circulation – as may be taken by the activities that come from electrical emanations about self – is helpful. But if these are passed as the equalizing from one extremity to another, and then the exercises, so much the better!" (681-2)

"Each day we would use the Radio-Active Appliance for one hour, attached to opposite sides of the body; right wrist, left ankle; left wrist, right ankle. This is to create – by the body-vibrations, that are brought to activative forces of forcing through the whole of the circulatory forces that renewal of energy and vitality – re-ionizing of the vital forces.

"After the treatment with the Radio-Active Appliance each day we would use a massage with an equal combination of Olive Oil and Tincture of Myrrh; that this may stimulate the circulation.

"These do, and keep activities cheery. Thus we may bring the better conditions for the body." (1384-2)

Occasionally, a body can be too ionized, as in this case:

"However, as we find, that needed instead of RE-ionizing is rather DE-ionizing of the vibratory forces of the body, for the better conditions." (1297-2)

Again, more information on the Radio-Active Appliance is coming in the Therapies chapter but for now know that it has nothing to do with nuclear energy. It is more like a radio wave device than nuclear fission!

—Carbon in the Blood—

"[We need] the active forces of carbon, or oxygen through the decomposed carbon, electrified, released IN the system – so as to re-VITALIZE the energies in the blood-stream." (5645-1)

"The body needs rest, mentally and physically, and the outside, open air, plenty of carbon – oxygen for the system – so that the blood supply is re-*ironized* throughout. Plenty of those food values that carry much of iron and iodine, reducing potashes in the system, as to relieve nerve tension." (5554-2)

Later in the section on Carbon Foods, this will be explained more fully. And "potashes" are associated with *potassium*, particularly certain types of potassium. Although it is an important mineral for the body, too much or too little potassium is known to result in cardiac arrhythmias.

The Often Forgotten *Lymph!*

For Cayce, and for most health care people, the human lymph system plays an important role in health. It is a circulatory system without the pump of the heart that the blood system enjoys. To move lymph one needs to – you guessed it – *MOVE!* Exercise the body is how the lymph gets moved along its many pathways and cleansing stations.

Here is just one of Cayce's comments on the importance of this system:

"There are ducts and glands and lymph throughout, both internally and externally, when these become impoverished by the lack of circulation in same it produces an inflammatory condition. Hence if we would build up the resistances in the blood stream by a greater quantity of lymph, these will take on the lymph first - for it is the white portion or the watery portion. Lymph flows through the lymph ducts and lymph glands, and is a part of the whole nerve circulation. Hence in the superficial portions it expresses or manifests itself in networks over all portions of the abdomen, through the groin, and works through those activities along the mammary glands and salivary glands, and all portions of the alimentary canal." (264-55)

The lymphatic system is an interconnected network of tissues and organs that play a key role in ridding the body of toxins, waste, and other undesirable materials. The primary function of the lymphatic system is to transport its special fluid containing infection-fighting white blood cells, the leukocytes and lymphocytes throughout our bodies.

The lymphatic vessels are connected to lymph nodes that filtered out elements in our system that need to be flushed away. The tonsils, adenoids, spleen and thymus are major parts of the lymphatic system. In our bodies there are hundreds of lymph nodes located deep inside our bodies. Many are around our lungs and heart, and many closer to the surface of our bodies – under our arm, in our groin, throat, and the like.

A lymphocyte is a type of leukocyte or white blood cell. White blood cells are the warriors in our bodies helping to fight off infection and cleanse dross away. Lymphocytes are the cells that determine the immune *response* to infectious microorganisms and alien substances. Lymphocytes compose roughly 20 to 40 percent of the total number of white blood cells in an adult body. They are concentrated in central lymphoid organs and tissues, such as the spleen, tonsils, and lymph nodes, as well as circulating through lymphatic vessels. These are the zone and pathways where our immune response will begin! The two primary types of lymphocytes are B-lymphocytes and T-lymphocytes, or you may have heard of B-cells and T-cells, especially T-cells because they became famous when the AIDS virus attacked humans. B- and T-cells originate from stem cells in our bone marrow. Some lymphocytes migrate to the thymus gland, where they mature into the important T-cells. These cells form what is called "immunologic memory." Such memory helps us to have a more rapid and vigorous response to a second encounter with the same toxin or other foreign substance that invades our body by the production of antibodies. This is how injections of small amounts of virus into our system can build antibodies against any future invasion. The ability to respond to virtually any toxin or alien substance comes from the massive variety of lymphocyte populations that our body contains, each of them with a receptor capable of recognizing a unique toxin or invader – any substance that is "not self" is attacked.

Keeping the lymph system moving and cleansed is an important part of health and healing. Exercise, water intake, massage, and hydrotherapies are some of the ways we keep our lymph flowing and ready to protect us. We will also see how maintaining an alkaline chemistry in our body helps the lymph fight infections and reduce toxins.

—The Nerves—

"As the electrical vibrations are given, know that Life itself, to be sure, is the Creative Force or God, yet its manifestions in man are electrical, or vibratory. Know then that the force in nature that is called electrical or electricity is that same force you worship as Creative or God in action!

"Seeing this, feeling this, knowing this, you will find that not only does the body become revivified, but by the creating in every atom of its being the knowledge of the activity of this Creative Force or Principle as related to spirit, mind, body, all three are renewed." (1299-1)

"We find the nerve system over-taxed and the body assimilating fear rather than stimulus of the nature to give relief to the body." (4790-1)

—Life is Electrical—

"The study of electrical energies is the basis for finding in a scientific manner the motivative force of animation in matter. ... But in the study of this activity of electronic energy in man, look for it in the *lower* frequency and not in the ultra. ... For Life is, and its manifestations in matter are of an *electronic* energy. (440-20)

"Materiality or matter demonstrates and manifests the units of positive and negative energy, or electricity, or God. Life itself is the Creative Force or God, yet its manifestations in man are electrical, or vibratory. Whatever electricity is to man, that's what the power of God is. Man may in the material world use God-force, God-power or electricity, to do man's work or to destroy himself. Know then that the force in nature that is called electrical or electricity is that same force you worship as Creative or God in action!" (1299-1)

—The Electrical Body—

"Electricity is life in the nerve force of the body. Impressions produced through the sensory system act on the nervous system of the body. Relays of these are along the stations of ganglia or nerve centers along the spine and in the deeper nervous system. The relays of nerves to the sensory system are through the sympathetics (autonomic system). Those of the cerebrospinal system, or the spinal cord, are in the brain itself, or the ends through the oblongata.

"Electrical forces from direct current will produce exaggeration or inflammation to the nerve walls. The reverse, or a cold electrical force, that is of low origin, produces a sullen, or acts as a sedative to the nerve force of the body. When we use electrical force in the nervous system, it should be of low origin or of cold storage or batteries applied along to the centers of the lymphatic circulation, to the armpits, ankles, or knee, and under them. Or the reverse current from static electricity along the spine or cerebrospinal forces. Add to this a positive suggestion to the mind as it goes to sleep, and will reach the sensory system by touch and hearing. Seeing this, feeling this, knowing this, you will find that not only does the body become revivified, but by the creating in every atom of its being the knowledge of the activity of this Creative Force or Principle as related to spirit, mind, body – all three are renewed. For these are as the trinity in the body, these are as the trinity in the principles of the very life force itself – as the Father, the Son, the Spirit – the Body, the Mind, the Spirit – these are one. One Spirit, One God, One Activity. Electricity is life; life is electricity, you see. Force or the power here in the atom in itself, which is the body drawn up, we have the electric force on the body will, if given into the nervous system, produce a reaction on the nerves themselves." (131-1)

—**The Electrical Poles of the Body**—

Electrical current is a complicated subject but let's take a moment to understand electrical current inside our bodies. First, here is Cayce's statement:

"The liver and the kidneys are the positive and negative poles of a human body, and when one of these becomes overtaxed, the other becomes supercharged in its functioning. Now, as to the activities of the liver and the kidneys, they are as the poles of a generator that are positive and negative in their reaction. The liver is an excretory and secreting organ. The kidneys are excretory and secreting, but in the opposite way and manner. The liver prepares values for the *assimilating*, and necessary elements to produce better assimilation. The functioning of the kidneys is rather to *purify* the circulation by taking from the blood supply infectious forces that are carried off by the slushing of same with the quantities of water taken. See?" (514-4)

In this teaching Cayce is showing how the current flows in our bodies. He is showing how the liver flows *to* the body giving that necessary for life while the kidneys draw *from* the body reducing toxicity by decomposing chemical compounds. This is a complementary process that keeps the body healthy.

He may also be touching on the process of electrolysis and bodily electrolytes, giving off and receiving electrons – see page 50 for more on electrolytes.

—Re-Ionizing the Nerve Forces—

"We find that there is the lack of ionization of the nerve forces, owing to the great strain that has been put upon the whole of the nervous system, as well as the manner of the circulatory system. Yet, these may be aided in creating a better coordination between the superficial and deeper circulation, and a better reaction or activity through the assimilating forces of the body." (1553-1)

Be sure to read his hot-and-cold shower therapy for improving superficial and deeper circulation on page 142.

"Q: Would breathing exercise for re-ionizing the system together with the head-and-neck exercise be well at this time?

"A: Not until we get the body coordinating better physically and physically-mentally. Then these exercises would be very well." (1523-17)

It is important for us to notice that Cayce is revealing the stages in healing. One must first get the coordination going before any exercise will be truly helpful.

"The electric forces [will] re-ionize the body-vitality. This would be of the low forms of electrical vibration as from the low static vibratory influence, rather than the direct currents." (1472-8)

The use of an electric massage vibrator was often recommended in Cayce's discourses. See page 146.

"[We need] re-ionizing or re-vitalizing or re-charging – as it were – the whole vital forces of the body itself ... to bring much better and much nearer NORMAL coordination." (1038-1)

"Use those vibrations as may be set up by the Radio-Active Appliance as may be attached to the body for the attuning or ionizing or re-electrifying of the energies of the system." (1125-2)

More information on the Radio-Active Appliance is coming in the Therapies chapter but for now you should know that despite this device's name it has nothing to do with nuclear energy. The name is associated with a radio rather than a radioactive nuclear device!

—Carbonizing the Nerve Forces—

"The body itself, the whole body, is not in as good condition to rebuild as we have had before, because we find the carbon of the body, or the storage battery of the body, which we have of course in the nerve tissue in the gray and white matter, is below par and below normal. Hence, the body is in a good deal worse condition that we have had." (5707-1)

We are carbon-based lifeforms. Here is famous physicist Stephen Hawking: "What we normally think of as 'life' is based on chains of carbon atoms, with a few other atoms, such as nitrogen or phosphorus."

White matter affects how the brain learns and functions. Grey matter is associated with information processing and cognition. White matter regulates the distribution of potential actions, playing the role a relay receiving and passing on information and messages, and coordinating communication between different brain regions.

How Mr. 5707, a twenty-year-old Texas boy, let his body become so low on energy is a bit of a mystery because carbon is found in nearly every food and provides energy to survive. Whatever foods you bite into you are sure to get plenty of carbon because carbon is present in most every food we eat! In this young man's reading Cayce's amazing mind saw this:

"The body has wasted away a good deal since we had him before, he is very thin; the blood is right thin. The building properties of the blood are rather below normal. The white blood is in the supremacy, and is different from what we had before, but the building tissue in the blood, which goes with the white and red blood both, is very weak, and we find the effects of it more through the lungs and through the larynx.

Also find the lower parts of the right lung very much involved; have a choking up of the tissue of the cells of the lung, but find no broken tissue there, though there are tubercular cells in two places." (5707-1)

Notice how tuberculosis may be the cause! Here is how Cayce sought to repair this young man's body, and notice how holistic his approach, being physical and mental:

"We will have to get the digestive organ in proper shape to have assimilations from the body. We must have more oxygen so that the lungs will throw off the carbon [carbon dioxide] from the body. He should be more out doors, and take more bodily exercise; have more employment of the mind, to get it off of self, or to do something that will relax the body – not enough of course to wear it out, causing congestion. Then the body will rebuild."

This gives us an idea of how complex healing and health is, and yet may be summed: digestion and assimilation of nutrients needed, elimination of toxins that build up in the body, and a mind that seeks to live and engage in fellowship (not being so self-centered). By the way, Edgar Cayce's wife developed tuberculosis and was cured using Cayce's methods.

—The Glands—

"All the elements for revivifying, or for producing reproduction of functioning of organs, activities, nerve forces, *are produced by glands*. Hence, the condition has been and is dependent upon the resuscitating of the influences [of the glands]. Hence the stimulation necessary along the cerebrospinal system, and the adjustments, as to allow the perfect flow of activity through the nerve impulses of ganglia activity. And, as the system is builded for better general health in assimilation, in distribution, it will aid the glands in producing or performing their necessary functions." (360-4)

"There must be those attentions to the body that will change the chemical reactions in which the glandular system takes from the body-forces, or the diet in the assimilation, to create the supplying elements for resuscitating and revivifying of the affected areas." (3543-1)

More detail on the glands will be coming the next chapter, particularly the endocrine glands for they are of major importance in Cayce's teachings for health and renewal.

—Coordination—

When Cayce was giving a health reading for a person his mind could actually "see" inside their body and he would usually go through in a sequence beginning with the blood supply, then the nervous system, onto the organs, and also adding in the person's emotional, mental state as well. His most common suggestions for improvement almost always included improving the eliminations and getting spinal manipulation and massage, and dietary changes. Rejuvenation and health came when the body's circulation and nerve flow were cooperating, as in this comment to a 41-year-old man:

"Circulation will then be reestablished, nerve flow and energies from all the centers through which the associations and connections between cerebrospinal and sympathetic nerves receive their impulses, must be rejuvenated, revivified." (3275-1)

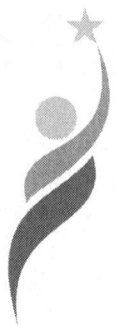

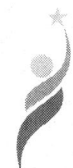

Chapter 5
The Glands and Our Two Nervous Systems

Edgar Cayce saw the glands in the human body as channels through which our souls incarnate.

Here is Edgar Cayce's extraordinary teaching in reading 281-38:

"The glandular forces then are ever akin to the sources from which, through which, the soul dwells within the body." And he expands on this, saying, "It may be easily seen, then, how very closely the glands are associated with reproduction, degeneration, regeneration; and this throughout—not only the physical forces of the body but the mental body and the soul body."

As we've just read, deterioration of bodily functions has a lot to do with the glandular secretions or lack there of, and the rejuvenation must also include improvements in glandular secretions. Of course, these "secretions" are the powerful hormones that affect bodily functions and chemistry.

Depending how you count them, the human body has roughly seven *endocrine* glands. "Endocrine" refers to glands that secrete hormones or other products *directly into the blood*. They are considered to be a "system," and are most often referred to as the Endocrine System.

I realize that most of us do not want or need to become Endocrinologists, but having some basic knowledge of this most important system in our body will help us in our efforts to gain and maintain health. Let's explore them:

—Hormones—

Hormones control the body's metabolism, growth, sexual development and functionality. When the hormones leave the glands they enter the bloodstream and are transported to organs and tissues in every part of the body.

—Endocrine Gland: Locations & Influence—

Here are the major endocrine glands in the body beginning in the lower torso and proceeding through the body to brain:

Ovaries and Testicles (Gonads)

The ovaries are located on either side of the uterus in females and secrete the hormones estrogen and progesterone; these hormones ensure sexual development, fertility and healthy menstrual periods. The testicles in males are located in the scrotum below the penis and secrete androgens, mainly testosterone, that control sexual development, puberty, facial hair, sexual behavior, libido, erectile function, and the formation of spermatozoa (spermatogenesis).

Cells of Leydig (Lyden)

The Leydig cells are located in the testes and release a male sex hormone called testosterone. These cells are also found in a woman's ovaries. They are named after their discoverer Franz Leydig, an anatomist from Germany. Also known as *interstitial cells of Leydig*, they play a vital role in maintaining proper levels of male hormones. When Leydig cells are exposed to Luteineizing Hormone (LH), which is secreted by the pituitary gland, they produce androgens, or male hormones. Inside the Leydig cells of *human* males can be found Reinke's crystals, small rod-shaped crystals made of protein. They occur only in humans and seem to occur in larger quantities in older men, leading some to believe that they are a byproduct of a degenerative process related to aging.

Adrenal glands (suprarenal glands)

These are located on top of the kidneys. These glands secrete corticosteroids and catecholamines, such as norepinephrine and adrenaline (epinephrine), which are hormones that are released *in response to stress*. These glands also produce aldosterone that affects kidney function.

Pancreas

Located in the abdomen the pancreas is both an endocrine gland and a digestive organ. It produces insulin, somatostatin, glucagon, and pancreatic polypeptide. Insulin plays a key role in carbohydrate and fat metabolism in the body. Somatostatin regulates endocrine and nervous system function; it inhibits the secretion of several hormones, such as gastrin, insulin and growth hormone. Glucagon is a peptide hormone that raises blood glucose levels when they fall too low. Pancreatic polypeptide helps control the secretion of substance. A peptide is a molecule that is made up of at least two amino acids.

Thymus gland

An endocrine gland located beneath the breastbone (sternum). T-cell lymphocytes, types of immune cells, mature and multiply in the thymus gland early in life. After puberty the gland shrinks. The thymus gland plays a role in the body's immune system.

Thyroid gland

It is located just below the Adam's apple in the neck; it produces hormones that play a key role in regulating blood pressure, body temperature, heart rate, metabolism, and how the body reacts to other hormones. The thyroid gland uses iodine to manufacture hormones. The two main hormones are thyroxine and triiodothyronine, which affects almost every physiological process in the body, including growth and development. The thyroid gland also produces calcitonin, which stimulates bone cells to add calcium to bone, as well as regulating calcium metabolism.

Parathyroid glands

Small endocrine glands located in the neck. They produce parathyroid hormone, which regulates calcium and phosphorous in the blood, blood clotting, and neuromuscular excitation.

Pineal body (pineal gland)

It is a pea-size gland located in the epithalamus, near the center of the brain, between the two hemispheres. It produces melatonin, a serotonin derived hormone, which affects the modulation of sleep patterns in both seasonal and circadian rhythms (physical, mental, and behavioral changes that follow a roughly 24-hour cycle, responding primarily to light and darkness in an organism's environment). Its shape resembles a tiny pinecone (hence its name).

Hypothalamus

This gland is located just above the brain stem, below the thalamus. This gland activates and controls involuntary body functions, appetite, sleep, temperature, as well as the circadian cycles. The hypothalamus links the nervous system to the endocrine system via the hypophysis (i.e. pituitary gland).

Pituitary gland

An endocrine gland located just off the hypothalamus at the base of the brain ("*hanging*" off of the hypothalamus). It is known as the "master gland," because it secretes hormones that regulate the functions of other glands, as well as growth and several body functions.

The anterior pituitary secretes hormones that affect sexual development, thyroid function, growth, skin pigmentation, and adrenocortical function – which enables the adrenal glands to deal with stress from every possible source, ranging from injury and disease to work and relationship problems. They largely determine the *energy* used in our body's responses to every change in our internal and external environment.

The posterior pituitary secretes oxytocin, a hormone that raises uterine contractions as well as ADH (antidiuretic hormone) that encourages the reabsorption of water by the kidneys.

—Summary—

In this attempt to simplify and summarize the hormones and glands (and at the risk of upsetting some Endocrinologists) we should understand that our body is a body-mind-spirit whole, so systemic activity in the body must take into consideration the mental attitude and emotional condition. Also, the Endocrine System operates as *a system*. Messages are going back and forth among the glands via the blood circulatory system – and rapidly! These hormonal messages affect health and wellbeing, energy, and rejuvenation, even moods and emotions, attitudes and motivations, or the lack thereof. And in turn they are affected by mental and emotional disposition.

Today, modern medicine is primarily pharmaceutical, meaning drug-therapy, and the approach is mostly toward stopping or reducing *symptoms* rather than *causes*. And though in some cases drugs are needed, returning the body to natural functioning using its own internal chemicals and processes should be the ultimate goal whenever possible.

Of course Cayce never left any discussion to the physical only, so we should take a moment and look into his spiritual comments about the glands:

—The Spiritual, Metaphysical Aspect of Glands—

Interestingly, the seven major zones of endocrine glands correlate well to the seven spiritual centers in the human body, often called "chakras." Here are the spiritual and metaphysical concepts associated with these glands:

Much of Cayce's insights into the glands were given in his series of readings numbered 281. The following is an example and I am leaving it in the format used for all of his readings to give you a better idea of how the files look:

"TEXT OF READING 281-53 This psychic reading given by Edgar Cayce at his home on Arctic Crescent, Virginia Beach, Va., this 2nd day of April, 1941, in accordance with request made by those present.

"PRESENT

"Edgar Cayce; Hugh Lynn Cayce, Conductor; Gladys Davis, Steno. Florence Edmonds, Esther Wynne, Frances Y. Morrow, Hannah Miller, Ruth LeNoir, Helen Ellington, Gladis Hardin, Sallie Jones, Mae Verhoeven.

"READING

"Time of Reading 3:55 to 4:20 P. M.

"1. HLC [Edgar's eldest son]: You will have before you the Glad Helpers Prayer Group, members of which are present in this room. You will consider their work and study on the endocrine system of the human body, answering the questions they submit, as I ask them:

"2. [Edgar Cayce]: Yes, we have the group gathered here; as a group and as individuals, also their work and study of the endocrine system in the human body, with the information which has been indicated through this channel - that was to be analyzed in the mind of each.

"3. Ready for questions.

"4. (Q) Are the following statements true or false? Comment on each as I read it: The life force rises directly from the Leydig gland through the Gonads, thence to Pineal, and then to the other centers.

"4. (A) This is correct; though, to be sure, as it rises and is distributed through the other centers it returns to the solar plexus area for its impulse through the system.

For the moment, let's consider the variation here in this life force - or as respecting this life force. The question is asked not in relation to the life alone as manifested in the human body, but as to the process through which coordination is attained or gained in and through meditation, see?

Hence physically, as we have indicated, there is first the nucleus - or the union of the first activities; and then the pineal as the long thread activity to the center of the brain, see? Then from there, as development progresses, there are those activities through reflexes to the growth or the developing of the body.

Interpret that variation, then, as being indicated here. One life force is the body-growth, as just described. The other is the impulse that arises, from the life center, in meditation.

"5. (Q) As the life force passes through the glands it illuminates them.

"5. (A) In meditation, yes. In the life growth, yes and no; it illuminates them in their own activity in life growth.

"6. (Q) The leydig gland is the same as that we have called the lyden, and is located in the gonads.

"6. (A) It is in and above, or the activity passes through the gonads. Lyden [See 281-53, R2] is the meaning - or the seal, see? while Leydig is the name of the individual who indicated this was the activity. You can call it either of these that you want to.

"7. (Q) The life force crosses the solar plexus each time it passes to another center.

"7. (A) In growth, yes. In meditation, yes and no; if there remains the balance as of the attunement, yes.

"When we are considering these various phases, the questions should be prepared so that they would not crisscross, or so that there would not be a confusion or a misinterpretation as to what is meant.

"You see, what takes place in the developing body, or in life growth (which we have used as a demonstration, or have illustrated), may be different from that which takes place as one attempts to meditate and to distribute the life force in order to aid another - or to control the influence as in healing, or to attain to an attunement in self for a deeper or better understanding. These questions or statements are such that they will be confusing to some; but if they are asked properly there will not be confusion.

"8. (Q) The solar plexus is the aerial gland.

"8. (A) No. By the term aerial we mean that impulse or activity that flows in an upward, lifting, raising or rising movement. It is an activity in itself, you see; not as a gland but as an activity UPON glands as it flows in, through, from or to the various centers of activity in the system itself. It is a function. Let's illustrate - possibly this will give an interpretation such that you may understand:

"In your radio you have what you call an aerial for communications that are without any visible connection. This is not a part of that making up the framework, yet it is necessary for certain characters of reception or for the better distribution of that which takes place in the instrument as related to communication itself.

"So in the physical body the aerial activity is the flow through the pineal, to and through all the centers. It aids the individual, or is an effective activity for the individual who may consciously attempt to attune, coordinate, or to bring about perfect accord, or to keep a balance in that attempting to be reached or attained through the process.

"As the process begins in the physical body, it is along the pineal; or it is the same movement that is the controlling or attuning influence from the mother with the developing forces of the body through the period of gestation.

"That is the manner, or the process, or the way in which the impressions are made. So, if there is beauty about the body of the mother through such periods, there are those influences to bring about accord. It may be indicated in contour of face. It may be indicated in the process of change in the activity of the thyroid as related to all the forces, - even to the color of hair or eyes, or the skin's activity; the nails, or more toes than should be - or less, or such activities. Or, the influences existent through such processes might make for a lacking of something in the body itself, pathologically; by the attempt to create a normal balance without the necessary influences being available.

"All of this is what we have referred to as the aerial activity, see?

"HLC: I see.

"Don't say you see if you don't see! You only had a portion of it! Let's illustrate it in this way, so you will comprehend:

"Understand the processes of activity through which there are the needs of the aerial in reception. For, of course, it is a matter of vibration in the body, as well as that illustrated in the physical condition. Thus there are activities about a body that is supplying the needs physically and mentally for a developing body, that become a part of the process, see?

"9. (Q) The entity preparing to be born into the earth has an influence upon the mother in building its own body.

"9. (A) No. That would be the same as saying that an atom had an influence upon that to which it could be attracted! See the variation?

"As in the realms outside of the material body, we have influences that are sympathetic one to another and we have influences that have an antipathy one for another, - as in fire and water, yet they are much alike. There are other forces that are active in the same manner, or that are of the

"But in the physical world there is builded a body, by the process of a physical law, see? Now: There is builded also a mental body, see?

"God breathed into man the breath of life and he became a LIVING soul.

"Then, with the first breath of the infant there comes into being in the flesh a soul, - that has been attracted, that has been called for, by all the influences and activities that have gone to make up the process through the period of gestation, see?

"Many souls are seeking to enter, but not all are attracted. Some may be repelled. Some are attracted and then suddenly repelled, so that the life in the earth is only a few days. Oft the passing of such a soul is accredited to, and IS because of disease, neglect or the like, but STILL there was the attraction, was there not?

"Hence to say that the body is in any way builded by an entity from the other side is incorrect. BUT those mental and physical forces that ARE builded ARE those influences needed FOR that soul that does enter!

"10. (Q) The entity desiring to enter governs the change in sex, which may occur as late as the third month.

"10. (A) It may occur even nineteen years after the body is born! So, it doesn't change in that direction!

"11. (Q) The physical development of the child is wholly dependent upon the mother from whom it draws physical sustenance, but its purpose, desire and hope are built up or influenced by the minds of all concerned.

"11. (A) That's the first question you've asked correctly. CORRECT!" (281-53)

See how Cayce fully understood the how the human body develops but then reinforces the influence of the mind, even the minds of all concerned.

The following is a reading given for Edgar Cayce himself, focusing on his psychic ability and the glands involved:

"(Q) What other glands in the body, if any, besides the Leydigian, pineal, and glands of reproduction, are directly connected with psychic development?

"(A) These three are the ducts, or glands. In some developments these have reached a stage where they do not function as ducts or glands, but are rather dormant; yet much passes through same, especially for the various stages of a psychical sojourn or development. These, as we find - the genitive organism is as the motor, and the Leydig as a sealed or open door, dependent upon the development or the use same has been put to by the entity in its mental, its spiritual, activity. The mental may have been misused, or used aright. The spiritual activity goes on just the same. It is as the electron that is Life itself; but raised in power and then misdirected may bring death itself, or - as in the activities of the glands as seen, or ducts - that used aright may bring serenity, hope, peace, faith, understanding, and the attributes of its source, as the experience of the entity; or, misdirected, may bring those doubts, fears, apprehensions, contentions, disorders, disruptions, in every portion of the body. Hence these may literally be termed, that the pineal and the Leydig are the SEAT of the soul of an entity.

"As to the abilities of physical reproduction, much of the activity of the Leydig makes for that as of embryonic in its activity, or of sterility in its activity. So we have those channels. These are not the psychic forces, please understand! They are the CHANNELS through which the activities have their impulse! Though the manifestations may be in sight, in sound, in speech, in vision, in writing, in dreams, in Urim or Thummim, or in any. For these represent Urim and Thummim in their essence, or in ANY of the RESPONDING forces in a body; but their impulse arises from or through these sources in much the same manner as the heart and the liver are of the physical body the motivating forces, or impulses, that carry the stream of life itself; or as the brain is that motivating center of impulse or mind. These are merely as illustrations that the student may better understand the activity of that being presented." (294-142)

As you can read, Edgar Cayce's vision saw us as spiritual beings living in physical vessels, and these two profoundly affect each other. And when the mind, which is the *bridge* between the physical and spiritual, is added to our composition, we have the whole self – what Cayce called "the entity."

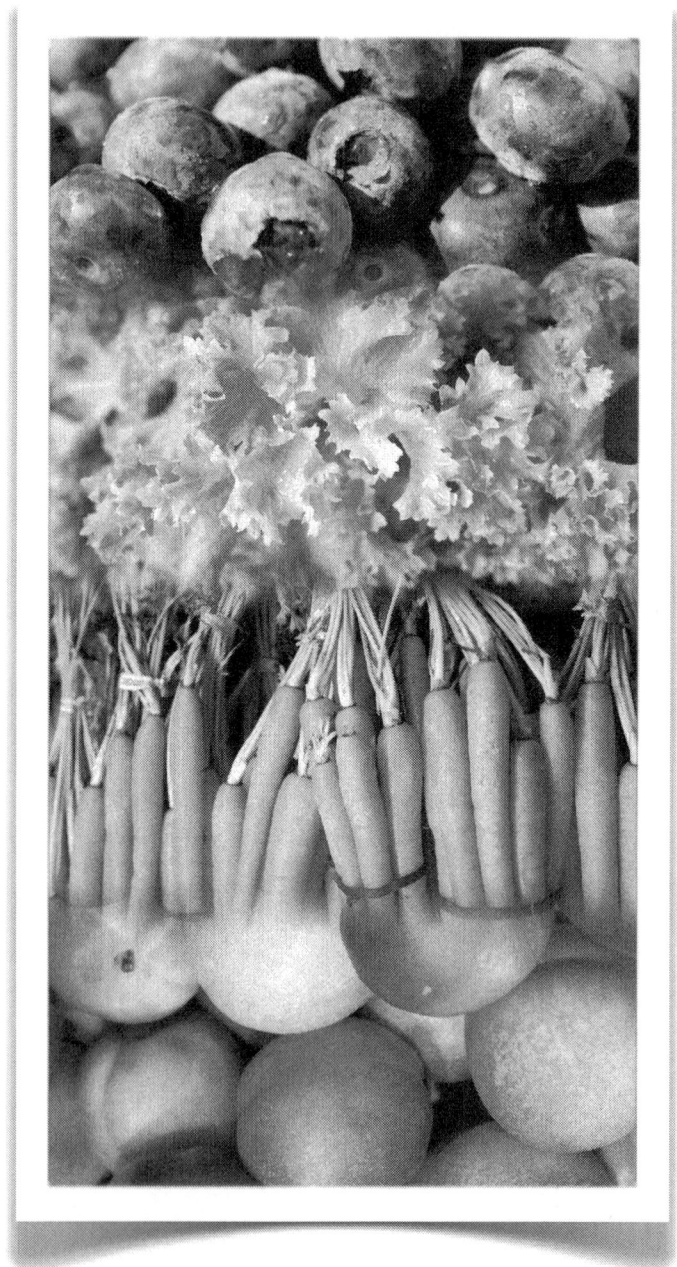

Fruits & Veggies

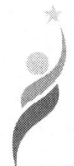

Chapter 6
Diet and Foods for Health & Healing

Edgar Cayce was preaching fruits and vegetables in the 1920s, '30s, and '40s to a meat-and-potatoes generation. He wanted more *raw* vegetables as well as cooked ones. And due to modern-day technologies for food growing and processing using pesticides, herbicides, preservatives, chemical and hormonal food additives, and more, we are far from the natural diet of our ancestors and those who live close to Nature. But we are much more conscious of this today and have many options for finding the right foods for our health and wellbeing.

Let's explore Cayce's many teachings about food.

—Blood and Nerve Building Foods—

"We would be mindful of the diet, that it consists principally of those of seafoods; of much that grows ABOVE the ground, as of the spinach, lettuce, and such GREEN vegetables. Any of the salads that carry large quantities of iron. Now this, apparently, would be the creating of blood, but blood of a character is needed." (5667-1)

"Do use a good deal of sea food, a great deal of leafy vegetables, and the character of foods that are body and blood building; as celery, lettuce, radish, carrots, beets, beet tops, watercress – all of these should be taken quite often; not every day, to become tiresome for the body, but these will be found to be most helpful." (3043-1)

"At present the diet would be those of the nature carrying the greater rebuilding forces in blood stream and in nerve tissue. Much then of green vegetable forces, and fish, that are necessary for the body's development. Little of those of starchy or of the heavy forces." (3837-1)

"There needs to be the care of the diet, for those conditions as necessary for the BUILDING of blood, of strength, of vitality, of muscle; and the body with this kind of food – not the highly seasoned, but that of the nutritious nature: Fish, fowl, and much vegetable; celery, lettuce, and the spring – or the vegetables green as much as possible. Cornbread (not white bread), whole wheat bread." (5618-5)

"In tomatoes there is found the three NECESSARY vitamins for growth and for DEVELOPMENT. The same is seen in carrots – save these are not BALANCED in the same ratio as in tomatoes – but THESE may be given in the raw state. With tomatoes, choose the well ripe (vine ripened). Another WELL balanced food with THIS ... is spinach, well cooked, with no oil or grease save butter. This will furnish another vitamin, an iron that is excellent for the blood. Well too that those of the glutens be used, which will be found by rolling wheat, raw wheat, see? and this cooked as a gruel – a little salt and little butter, and a very SMALL quantity of sugar." (5520-2)

To cook a porridge like "a gruel" means to keep it watery and thin, not letting it thickened by evaporating the water.

"In the matter of diet – these should be nerve and blood building, but do not force self to eat that as is not desirous of being eaten! Do not over STIMULATE the system with those of any character of foods that supply over abundance of sugars, or over abundance of alcoholic forces, as when there are those of fruits and fruit juices taken, do not take those that produce fermentations within the system; for these unbalance the ASSIMILATING forces of the system, as does over-acidity or too highly seasoned foods." (5423-1)

"Q: Are the sores on face caused from sugar in the blood?

"A: Rather from the lack of GLUTEN in the blood, that KEEPS the eliminating system in coordination. With the strengthening of the vitality of the nerve ends of the nervous system, with the stimuli to the glands of the body in every direction, we will find these conditions will disappear – but the WARNINGS, as given, do NOT take properties that make for too much sugars or too much of the stimuli in that of ACIDITY in the system." (5423-1)

"Fruits, vegetables are better, but not much of meats. One meal each day, whether morning, evening or in the noon, one whole meal should consist of RAW vegetables. Combine these of all the leafy and all those vegetables that may be combined in a salad. Lettuce, celery, carrots, beans, spinach, onions, cabbage, and or all of these. Such a salad may be changed occasionally to a whole FRUIT meal; as apples, oranges, peaches, lemons, pears – don't put in any bananas! All of these may be combined and used instead of the meal of vegetables. Meats if they are taken at all should never be fried; in fact, *no fried foods at all!*" (1204-2)

—Vitamins—

"Do add more strengthening foods to the body-forces in the diets which carry E vitamins as well as A and B or the B-complex or B-combinations, niacin and iron. For we must enrich the blood from the deteriorations that are beginning to indicate how a form of anemia is affecting the resistances of the body.

"Do follow the diets in foods which are rich in necessary minerals for replenishing blood supply. The E vitamin, the wheat germ with the cereals or wheat germ oil taken in capsule at least once a week or twice during the week. Best that it be varied, one week once a week, next week twice a week, next week three-times, but have regular periods for it. The B-1 should be rich in the foods which are taken. We would find this from all foods which are yellow in color, not as greens that would turn yellow, but as the yellow variety of squash, carrots, wax beans, peaches, all of these are well. Though, there are other foods, to be sure, as liver, beef juices, fish, all of these are well to be portions of the diet." (5319-1)

"The continual taking of such [B-complex vitamins] will do very little good, unless the system is so adjusted that these may be assimilated so that the strength and vitality may go into the system through glandular activity and be distributed through blood and nerve supply. When the corrections are made [adjustments to spine and reduction of toxins in system] these supplementary vitamins may be taken (not in the beginning) and assimilated by the body so as to gain strength." (5017-1)

—Ionizing and Ironizing Foods—

"Alternate between those foods that carry a large percentage of iron and those that carry assimilated ionized forces as with iodine. Or let most of the foods now be with fish, shell fish or the like." (1225-3)

"Q: Would you recommend any specific diet?

"A: The fresh vegetables, raw vegetables, are preferable to meats; for the body needs the balancing throughout the system of the centralizing system being kept ionized as related to the eliminations of the body." (865-1)

"Too much calcium in the system, too much potash, and not sufficient amount of iodine as related to the ironizing and oxidization as take place in the system." (51-1)

Cayce reference to too much calcium and too much potash is very interesting. Both of these are inorganic minerals (neither animal nor vegetable) in structure. They both form the ash when animal or plant materials are burned! The organic portions of burned animals or plants are gone, easily assimilated into the biosphere, but the ash remains. Apparently, Cayce would have us be more on the side of organic, easily assimilated condition – with ironizing and ionizing energies in the blood system rather than too much ash. As mentioned earlier, potash is a term associated with potassium, particularly certain types of potassium. Although it is an important mineral for the body, too much or too little potassium is know to result in cardiac arrhythmias. Sources of potassium are bananas, oranges, apricots, avocados, potatoes, bran, peanuts, and dried peas and beans. Sources of calcium are milk, cheese and seafoods (mussels, oysters, salmon, shrimp, etc.). Of course, these same seafoods also provide iodine. Perhaps Mr. 51 was ingesting too much of the milk and dairy sources of calcium without getting enough iodine.

"Change the diet, keeping the oils – not only the olive oil, but those of the cod-liver oil, to replenish the blood supply. IRONIZING the whole system, as it were." (5554-2)

—Carbon Foods—

Carbon is found in nearly every food and provides energy to survive. All foods contain carbon. Only water does not. During metabolism our bodies break the bonds between carbon molecules releasing energy that our cells can use.

Cayce seems to be using the term "carbon" in a manner similar to how we use "carbohydrate." However, in 5707-1, he does seem to be differentiating a true carbon food from a starchy carbon food. Carbohydrates [literally a combination of the words "carbon" and "water"] are formed from carbon, hydrogen, and oxygen through a complex process in which plants with green leaves transform energy from the sun. The plant uses some of the carbohydrate for its own needs; the rest is stored in various parts – seeds, leaves, stalks, roots, tubers, and so on. This stored carbohydrate can easily be broken down, digested, and assimilated into our systems. Carbohydrates in bread, pasta, and cereal need to be made from the *whole* grain. Carbs are also found naturally in fruits, berries, maple sap, honey, sugars (beet sugar is Cayce's preference) and milk.

There is a vast array of foods that contain carbohydrates. It appears that Cayce would prefer we use carbohydrates that do *not* contain sugars and starch, but yield a pure carbon influence when digested. When we study his recommended diet, it does *not* contain flour pastas and processed breads. It *does* contain whole-grain cereals, as well as fruits and vegetables. These would appear to be the better sources of carbon.

Here are some of his comments and directives:

"It is better for the body to eat oftener instead of in large quantities. He should not eat so much of a starch, but more of a property that will produce carbon to the body, so that it will not burn itself out." (5707-1)

"[We need] plenty of carbon, oxygen for the system, so the body can be re-ironized. Plenty of those food values that carry much of iron and iodine, reducing potashes in the system, as to relieve nerve tension." (5554-2)

"A diet of a nature of carbons to the system to rebuild or rejuvenate the blood forces. The iron and calcium into the system will produce more of a system to call fuel for the system." (4801-1)

Occasionally, the body has too much carbon, as in this case:

"Keep the diet in that way and manner that will produce at all times the easy digestion. Not too much of fuels or carbons, or carbohydrates, but more of the protein and vegetable forces that give the tissue in the white blood and lymphatic forces." (4988-2)

—The Acid and Alkaline Balance—

One of Cayce's frequent diet teachings was the advantage of a slightly alkaline body chemistry. The following are some of his comments on acid/alkaline balance in our diet. At the end of these comments is a list of foods and their influence in our bodies.

"As we have maintained for this body *and for others*, a tendency towards more of the alkalin-reacting foods; for when there is the tendency towards an alkalin system there is less effect of cold and congestion. Adhere to the alkalin reacting diets, that may be had from vegetables; and at least one meal, or one period each day, or at least two or three days apart, have those wholly raw. Have less of the sweets, or not too great a quantity. Naturally, there should be sweets that tend to make for the proper distribution of sugar for the system, for sugars - to be sure - supply not only heat but also the proper balance for proper fermentation, as do starches; but if these arise more from fruits and vegetables rather than the addition of cane sugar into the body, it will be much the better, for then less acidity arises from same. To be sure, there should be sufficient of starch and of the alkalin reactions to produce proper fermentation, or the proper character of the alcohol that is so necessary in the preserving the calorie content, in a manner; though the calories may be made too high, but the activity of the necessary vital forces that act with the hemoglobin and in the urea of the blood itself. Hence an alkalin diet, as has been indicated - or as may be indicated from charts of same, would be the correct way and manner. Do not have overeating at any time. Keep a well-balance. And, as some have very much commented on or maintained, if meats are to be taken in any quantity don't eat a lot of starch with same; if there's to be a lot of sweets taken, don't eat a lot of starch or proteins either with it; but keep them well-balanced." (270-33, my italics)

"In the matter of the diets: Here we need body-building foods, but those that tend to be more alkaline-producing than acid – for the natural inclinations of disturbed conditions in a body are to produce acidity through the bloodstream. Hence, we need to REVIVIFY same by the use of much of those that produce more of the enzymes, more of the hormones for the blood supply; yet not overburdening the body with those unless the balance in the vitamin forces is carried." (1302-1)

"Those that are blood and nerve building, and may be changed to any of the characters of foods that are ALKALINE

REACTING! Eggs may be taken at this time, provided the YOLK only is prepared, either in the form of hard and WELL MASHED afterward, mixed with any of the oils – olive oil, also those of cod-liver oil, should be part of the diet.

"Well that the irrigations of oil be occasionally used for the lower portion of the system, so that the colon may be cleansed properly, and that the STRAIN as has been induced by the lack of blood supply through this portion of the system may be increased. BUILD up the general system.

"The manipulations (osteopathic/chiropractic) as would be given in this condition would be for the strengthening of the whole nerve system, that the body may relax thoroughly when it rests – for the BUILDING properties for THIS body will be found in rest and sleep." (5520-2)

"Do set up the alkalinizing of body and the eliminations of poisons." (5319-1)

"As to the diet, keep more of the alkalines. No heavy foods that EVER are fried. And let one meal each day be of only raw green vegetables; not green in color necessarily, but in their very nature – those that carry all the vitamins necessary in creating the effluvia within the blood and nerve supply that is revivifying in its very nature." (743-1)

Researchers have found that cold germs and flu viruses and other diseases, such as cancer, need an acid environment in order to grow and thrive. Therefore, the goal for healthiness is to maintain a pH that is just slightly on the alkaline side. This is done by what many researchers refer to as the 80/20 rule in which 80 percent of the foods eaten are alkaline reacting, and 20 percent are acid reacting. The body functions optimally at an alkaline pH of approximately 7.35–7.45; any deviation just above or below this range can result in illness.

Here's a list of foods and their alkaline or acid forming influence in our bodies. It was prepared by HealingCancerNaturally.com/edgarcayce-nutritional-balance.html and I have added some commentary.

—Alkaline-forming fruits—

Apples, apricots, avocados, bananas, berries (all except blueberries and cranberries), cherries, citrus fruits like grapefruit, lemons, limes, oranges and tangerines, dates, figs, grapes, melons, papaya, passion fruit, peaches, pears, pineapples, pomegranates, tomatoes

—Alkaline-forming fruits—

Apples, apricots, avocados, bananas, berries (all except blueberries and cranberries), cherries, citrus fruits like grapefruit, lemons, limes, oranges and tangerines, dates, figs, grapes, melons, papaya, passion fruit, peaches, pears, pineapples, pomegranates, tomatoes

—Alkaline-forming grains—

Amaranth, millet, quinoa. All other grains are acid-forming.

—Alkaline-forming vegetables—

Alfalfa and other sprouts, Artichokes, Asparagus, Bamboo shoots, Beans, Beets, Bell Peppers, Broccoli, Brussels sprouts, Cabbage, Carrots, Cauliflower, Celery, Chard, Chicory, Collard greens, Corn, Sweet cucumber, Dandelion, Eggplant, Garlic, Kale, Kohlrabi, Leeks, Lettuce, Mushrooms, Mustard greens, Okra, Onions, Parsnips, Peas, Potatoes, Pumpkin, Radishes, Rhubarb, Sea vegetables, Spinach, Squashes, Watercress, Yams and Sweet potatoes.

—Alkaline-forming nuts—

Almonds, chestnuts and coconut, all others are acid-forming.

—Alkaline-forming, miscellaneous—

Agar-agar, apple cider vinegar, coffee, egg yolks, fruit juices, gelatin taken with fruit or vegetables, Glycothymoline, herbal teas, herbs fresh and dried, and most spices, honey raw (unpasteurized - and Cayce recommended it be in the honey comb) and mineral water.

—Alkaline-forming dairy—
Buttermilk fresh, milk - raw, whey, yogurt.

—Acid-forming fruits—
Blueberries, cranberries, plums, prunes and sulfurated dried fruits.

—Acid-forming vegetables—
There is much discussion of this topic and what should be listed here. Often legumes are list as acid-producing when there are exceptions and counter views to this. Here is the view of the Paleo Diet people (a diet based on the types of foods presumed to have been eaten by early humans): "Green beans, snow peas, green peas, and other green legumes encapsulated in pods are often questioned in the Paleo world. Are they Paleo? The short answer is yes, but here's why. When we say don't eat legumes, it's because legumes have certain anti-nutrients in them, like phytic acid and lectins. Phytic acid binds to the minerals magnesium, calcium, zinc, and iron in your gut and removes them, unabsorbed, from your body. And lectins are sticky little suckers that can glom onto your gut lining and wreak havoc on its integrity. Not good. However, nuts and seeds also contain these things, and you're still "allowed" to eat those on the Paleo diet. And that's because we're assuming you're not going to fill half your plate with nuts and seeds like you might with lentils or black beans. It's a quantity thing, and so it is with green beans and snow peas. Yes, those things contain those anti-nutrients, but if you're not eating them by the shovelful, you'll be just fine. Also, the greener the plant, the less phytic acid and lectins it contains. Green beans actually only contain trace amounts of phytic acid. And the lectins and the phytic acid are mostly found in the seed itself – not the pod. So

eat your green beans, snow peas, and even your green peas on occasion. Just don't make them a staple or a large proportion of your plate and you'll be just fine." (Source: paleoplan.com/2012/08-14/are-green-beans-and-snow-peas-paleo)

Usually found under acid-forming vegetables are dried beans, lentils, and chickpeas.

—Acid-forming Dairy—

Butter, cream, cheese, cottage cheese, milk pasteurized, homogenized, boiled, canned, dried.

—Acid-forming miscellaneous—

Alcoholic drinks, drugs (most prescription), egg whites, gelatin, soft drinks, tea (black), and tobacco. Some vegetable oils and vinegar. All meats, all fish.

Sometimes the body can become too alkaline, as in these readings:

"There has become an excess of alkalinity, and thus, through the digestive system, there is a lack of sufficient of the acids to produce proper digestions in the system." (3481-3)

Cayce wanted a slightly alkaline body for all of us but we should be aware that a body that is too alkaline is not good.

"(Q) What causes the body to vomit food at times?

"(A) As indicated, the excess of alkalinity." (462-6)

—**Climate Acclimation**—
Acclimate Yourself

We should consider one of Cayce's unusual tips for health and wellbeing: acclimating ourselves to the area in which we reside by eating vegetables and fruits grown in that area. Apparently, produce grown in our area contains qualities, vibrations, and "Nature codes" unique to our habit and these help our bodies adjust to our environment. By ingesting these, we better acclimate our bodies to the weather, air, water, pollens, vibrations, and "Nature codes" natural to our surroundings.

In reading 257-214, Cayce said, "Fruits, vegetables, grown wherever the body is active – especially leafy vegetables, and of those natures that supply the vital forces for energizing the system" are best. "Do not have large quantities of any fruits, vegetables, meats, that are not grown in the area where the body is at the time it partakes of such foods. This will be found to be a good rule to be followed by all. This prepares the system to acclimate itself to any given territory." (3542-1) The more often we eat "those foods or vegetables grown in the area where the body is residing, when practical," the better. (257-236) And he's not unrealistic about this, noting that "there are seasons that this becomes impractical, to be sure." But the principle of acclimation through ingestion of local foods is important and doable during the spring, summer, and fall season. He explains in 264-23: "In every clime where the atmosphere reactions are for a body, those vegetables grown in the immediate vicinity are much better than those grown in other places and prepared in any manner to be used by a body, see?"

So how do we do this? Well, there are two obvious ways: (1) plant our own garden and eat freshly picked foods from that garden; and (2) make connections with local farmers, farmers markets, and roadside food stands – and eating their locally grown foods.

—Local Farmers—

Many towns and cities now have Farmers Markets to which local or regional farmers bring their produce for sale. But ask the farmers where their farm is, because some will drive a long way to sell their produce. In my area, Virginia Beach, we have farmers from North Carolina selling at our local Farmers Market. Not that North Carolina wouldn't be considered "our area" when compared with produce from South America! Certainly some items from North Carolina would be fine.

You may be able to find local and regional farmers listed online.

Be alert. Watch out for local produce markets that *appear* to have locally grown produce but they are actually getting shipments from faraway places and selling them locally. This happens even at the local Farmers Markets. Ask them where their produce is *grown*. Amid the local produce is often produce from far, far away places with very different climates than yours.

If you're also interested in *organically* grown foods rather than those using chemical pesticides, herbicides, and chemical fertilizers, you'll have to look more carefully to find organic farmers. Though this is an up-and-coming trend, there may not be farms in your surrounding area that are organically growing their produce. And most chain grocery stores are selling "organic" produce from places with different climates than yours. This is another advantage in growing your own produce.

—Your Own Garden—

Growing your own garden can be as simple as growing a few plants in porch pots to tilling a large area of your backyard. It depends on your circumstances.

As noted in the reading I quoted earlier, Cayce would guide us to begin with "leafy vegetables, and of those natures that supply the vital forces for energizing the system." In Cayce's eyes, these would be "celery, lettuce, tomatoes, carrots, turnips, or any of these." You can begin by growing these indoors, in starter pots with "plant mixture," not plant soil. Plant mixture is specially designed for growing seeds into starter plants. Then when the weather is right and the seeds have developed some initial strength in root and tops, plant them in your own garden and they will grow conditioned to your environment.

—Local Gardeners—

Another resource for locally grown produce is gardeners! They often have more produce than they can use and would be happy to see it used rather than lost. Ask around about who is into gardening and if they have surplus to share. You may have to do little work to get this produce, such as pick your own, but it's worth it. And Cayce's readings say that it is very good for us to be out in the open, in the sunlight, among soil and vegetable growth. In some cases this garden produce is also grown without pesticides, herbicides, and chemical fertilizers. Unlike grocery stores, farms and gardens grow in coordination with Nature's growing cycle; so various produce gown locally is only available at different times of the seasons. For example, lettuce is early in the growing season and corn is later.

—Cayce's Ideal Diet—

One has to be careful how the Cayce readings on diet are presented, because many of his suggested diets were based on the condition and circumstances of the person seeking the reading. But if one studies enough of his readings, then the following diet appears to be a good, general diet for all.

Breakfast

Alternate the morning meal: One in which whole grains are the main course, and then another when eggs and/or fruits are the main course.

The morning with eggs and/or fruits, citrus fruits go well with the eggs but never with the grains. According to Cayce, citrus should never be taken at the meal with whole grain cereals or milk. Reserve the citrus for the egg breakfast. Interestingly, Cayce did recommend that dark-bread toast (pumpernickel, and the like) could be taken on the same morning as the citrus. Curiously, he recommended that with oranges or orange juice, one should add a few drops of lemon. With grapefruits or grapefruit juice, one should add a few drops of lime. I have no idea why this is the case. He also allowed us to have *crisp* bacon on these egg mornings. He was very insistent about it being *crisp*; in some cases he actually said "*very* crisp bacon" but not burned.

His most commonly recommended way for eggs to be cooked was *coddled*, something very few people do today. A coddled egg is one that is cooked more gently, slowly, and lightly than a boiled egg. It results in a more tender egg than the hard-boiled method. Coddle an egg just long enough so that the white is set but the yellow yolk is still soft and runny. The two methods for coddling an egg are cooked in the shell or cooked in a coddling dish. The difference between a soft-boiled egg and a coddled egg is that one is cooked in boiling water while the other is cooked slowly in simmering water. This method was quite popular in the 1920s and '30s with the use of the "eggcup." The earliest record of eggcups was found in 3 AD in the ruins of the city of Pompeii. After the fall of classical civilization in the east (1453 AD) and the west (476 AD), the eggcup would not be used again until the Elizabethan period of the 1600s. During this time, the ruling classes of England would often eat their eggs in silver eggcups.

Today one may use an egg cooker using steam to cook the egg in its shell.

Another unique Cayce perspective is that the whites of eggs create acidity in our bodies, whereas the yolks generate alkalinity; therefore, he often recommended that we eat the yolk and less of the whites, in some cases, none of the whites. This is in direct contrast to modern day teachings in which many people eat so-called "heart healthy" eggs that are whites only!

Again, the egg breakfast could also include "stewed fruits or baked apples, or things of that nature." (677-2) But more often he recommended citrus fruits when having the egg breakfast.

On the morning of the whole-grain cereal breakfast he sometimes recommended cooking as hot cereal and at other times as cold cereal, even at times as a "dry cereal". He said that *puffed* whole grain cold cereals were the better choice (such as puffed wheat). However, today most puffed whole grain cereals are covered with a sweetener! For some he approved the addition of bananas, but others were told never to add them to their cereals. For some, raisins were allowed, for others he discouraged them, explaining that raisins changed the influence of the cereal upon their bodies. Steel cut oats or whole wheat were suggested. Whether this was in opposition to rolled oats is unclear. But he was very clear about not combining citrus with cereal. Milk could be added to cereal, but in several readings he recommended adding a little butter and salt rather than milk and/or sugar.

When it came to sugar, Cayce was not insensitive to some people's need to sweeten certain meals. However, he recommended that we move away from cane sugar toward beet sugar, indicating that it was easier on the body. He also mentioned brown sugar (which is a less refined and more moist than plain cane sugar) and saccharin for people who shouldn't take much or any sugar (diabetics). Here's his comment on saccharin: "This should be good for the body, for it supplies more of the carbons in the system, and is the active principle of sweet that forms the basis of the active forces in the gastric juices, as termed, for those of proper fermentation in the system, and it is better than those that come of cane, corn, or of others, save the conditions wherein the sweets from BEET are better than saccharin." (255-3) Honey was also a good alternative to sugar. (1188-10)

Locally grown grains are going to be hard to find. But locally grown chickens and their eggs may be easier than you imagine. Of course, depending upon where you live, citrus may be nearby or far away. We could say that East Coast people should use Florida citrus and West Coast people California citrus. There's going to be some degree of local acclimation with that plan. Note that Cayce said: "Florida oranges carry more iron than those grown in California, while those of the southern states, or in the Rio Grande valley, carry more than those even in Florida." (255-3)

Lunch

This was the meal that Cayce often recommended to be totally raw vegetables. Hence, this is the meal for locally grown produce. Apparently, the juices in these raw vegetables are very good for our bodies. "Have raw vegetables during the noon portion of the day." (1137-1) He often recommended that we maintain a specific ratio between the number of vegetables that we eat which grow above ground to those that grow below ground. That ratio was 3 above ground to every 1 grown below ground. There were times when he changed this ratio to 5 to 1. But 3 to 1 was the most frequently recommended. In one reading, he actually added a list of below ground vegetables that could be considered to be *above ground*: "Such vegetables as turnips, parsnips, beets, carrots or radishes may be included among those grown *above* the ground." (677-2) His most commonly recommended vegetables were the "leafy green" ones.

Gelatin salads were also mentioned. Broths and soups were occasionally recommended as well.

Dinner

"Have a well-balanced cooked vegetable diet for the evening meal, using three vegetables grown above the ground to one grown below; with lamb, fowl or fish." (1137-1) This quote reflects Cayce's most common recommendation for the evening meal. He did occasionally recommend liver, usually no more than once a week. As far as acclimation is concerned, fish may well be found locally in rivers, streams, lakes, and bodies of water near where you live. In some areas you will be able to get fowl that has been raised fairly close by.

Here's one of his discourses listing his commonly suggested diet.

"As to the matter of diet, this would be a general outline that may be altered as the need arises:

"Mornings - citrus fruit juices, stewed fruits or cereals, with rice cakes, coddled egg, occasionally crisp bacon if desired; not a great amount of coffee or tea, and do not use the citrus fruit juices AND the cereals at the same meal - but alternate; and these will keep a normalcy.

"Noons - green vegetables, or vegetable juices made from fresh vegetables - or from vegetables that may be combined to make such juices. These will keep a normal balance in there actions to the assimilating system.

"Evenings - a well balanced diet of well cooked vegetables or meats. Lamb, fowl or such are well. Not too much meats or of any flesh that is fried, whether fish or fowl or animal meat; rather these should be broiled or well cooked in roasts or the like.

"As we find, these will keep a well balance and bring about the abilities - in the reactions of the body, in the physical and mental forces - for much bettered conditions." (437-6)

As we now see, he was quite consistent in his diet recommendations.

Let's look at his comments on specific food groups.

—Vegetables—

"For this body, eat more vegetables grown above the ground than those below the ground. Each day, though, have at least two or three raw vegetables; whether celery, lettuce, tomatoes, carrots, turnips, or any of these. These may be grated together and combined with a salad dressing that is of an olive oil base." (1217-2)

Freshness was important to Cayce:

"From the fresh vegetables, they should combine all those of the leafy nature; though not necessarily all at one time; and carrots, turnips, parsnips and the like; tomatoes, okra, and such natures - when they are cooked in their fresh state. When juices are taken that have already been prepared in their various combinations, they should be especially of celery, spinach, lentils, leeks, and such natures; and these may be combined with those that are the more easily obtained fresh, that are usually cooked together." (437-6)

Here's another:

"Use those foods that are nerve and blood building, that we may find in the fresher, greener vegetables given in whatever form is palatable to the body. But eat as much celery and lettuce, especially, as the body may consume at ANY time. Keep these; and know that through the Creative Energies that are manifested in a material world - in the prayers to the All-Wise Creative Energy or Force we worship as God, there may be brought BLESSINGS into the experience of those that labor with and for the development of a physical body, that this soul may manifest in this material world." (735-1)

In come cases Cayce recommended a purely fresh vegetable meal, as in this reading:

"We would have one meal each day, whether noon or evening, consisting almost entirely - or including mostly - of the raw fresh vegetables. These may be taken in the form of a salad or the like. Combine especially such as lettuce, celery, with whatever other vegetables the body may desire; as peppers or tomatoes, carrots, beets, turnips - if these are all grated when they are prepared, it would be preferable; or mustard. Any or all of these are well. Red Cabbage especially, if this is grated very fine and prepared with the others, raw, would be well. An oil or a salad dressing may be used. All of these would not be used at once, of course, but as many as may be eaten combined at one meal during the day would be well." (1654-1)

Here's another:

"In the diet, at least have a raw vegetable in the meals during each day. Such a salad may be composed of any or all of these: tomatoes, lettuce, celery, onions, radish, leeks, or mustard and the like; or slaw, celery, cabbage, or any or all of these." (437-8)

—Cooking Vegetables in Patapar Paper—

In over a hundred readings Cayce encouraged us to cook our vegetables in their own juices using Patapar paper (a parchment paper that seals in vitamins and minerals). You can buy Patapar paper on Amazon.com and Baar.com. Here are 3 examples:

"The preferable way to prepare such [vegetable] juices would be through cooking the vegetables after tying them in Patapar paper; not putting them in water to boil, but cooking either in the Patapar paper or in a steam steamer, so that only the juices from the vegetables may be obtained - and no water added in the cooking at all. Then these juices should be combined and seasoned to the taste. Even these vegetables and the chicken or fish would be better cooked in the Patapar paper." (133-4)

Steam cookers and little steaming trays or racks that fit into the bottom of any pan with boiling water in it and keep the veggies out of the water are sold most everywhere. I found a stainless steel rack for $3. It fits into my regular sauce pan.

"The vegetables that are taken should be preferably cooked in their OWN juices, as in Patapar paper. This will make a vast difference in the building of resistance." (861-1)

"If [vegetables are] cooked in Patapar paper they would be found to be more digestible - and only season with a little salt, pepper and butter." (357-7, he only wanted red pepper, not black)

—Fruits—

"Take plenty of citrus fruits and citrus fruit juices, and also the whole grain cereals - as the whole grain of oats or wheat, or a combination of wheat and barely (as in Maltex or the like). DO NOT have the fruits AND the cereals at the same meal, however. Alternate these, having the citrus fruits three or four mornings a week - as the orange juice, grape fruit, pineapple, lemons or the like; and then having the cereals the other mornings, and so on." (2432-2)

Here's another:

"Fruits such as canned pears, canned peaches or the like, provided these are not canned with benzoate of soda [often labeled Sodium Benzoate, and used as a preservative in many products]. Plums and others may be included in such a salad." (257-129)

And another:

"Let the food values be rather, as given, fruits - citrus fruits, grapes, pears, no bananas or apples. Any other fruits may be taken; plums or peaches, or those that are canned in peaches or apricots, so there is no benzoate of soda or a preservative in those used. Those that are used should be not the syrup so much but the fruit itself may be taken occasionally." (773-4) Today we can buy canned fruits in fruit juice only, no syrup. Again one has to be careful about additives, especially preservatives. Read the labels.

When it came to apples Cayce was not a fan of eating raw apples, rather baked apples where his preference, and those varieties that have the "bumps" or lobes on their under side. He also wanted apples to be eaten alone, without other foods at the same time.

In the case of bananas Cayce was also cautious, occasionally stating clearly to not eat them while at other times allowing them, even on cereal in the morning. In one reading he said bananas could only be eaten if tree-ripened! Well no bananas are available that have not been taken off the tree in their green state – a state in which the fruit has not released its natural sugars yet. But again, bananas from his perspective were better eaten alone, without other foods.

—Dairy—

There are many opinions about dairy products, and I cannot cover them all, so do some research and some experiments with your own body to learn how various dairy products react in your system.

Here are some of Cayce's comments regarding dairy products:

"There is so easily an over-stressing upon milk, by many; for there are many products much more healthful than milk. So few milks are free from tubercle; so few are free from those influences that cause a great deal more irritation than help - unless irradiated or dried milk is used. These [irradiated or dried milk] as a whole are much more healthful to most individuals than raw milk." (480-42)

In the reading you just read Cayce is referring to tubercle bacilli in cows' milk as a possible source of tuberculosis disease in humans. Keep in mind that the tuberculosis epidemic in North America was between 1800 through 1940 – during the period of Cayce giving health advice. Between 1912 and 1937 some 65,000 people died of tuberculosis contracted from consuming milk in England and Wales alone. By 1930 over 500 cities in the United States mandated pasteurization. In 1947 states began to require full pasteurization of milk, and the federal government prohibited the interstate sale of raw milk.

French scientist Louis Pasteur invented pasteurization. In 1864 Pasteur discovered that heating beer and wine was enough to kill most of the bacteria that caused spoilage, preventing these beverages from turning sour. The process achieves this by eliminating pathogenic microbes and lowering microbial numbers to prolong the quality of the beverage. Today, pasteurization is used widely in the dairy industry and other food processing industries to achieve food preservation and food safety. Pasteurization is not sterilization. Sterilization means the complete destruction of all microbic life. This is not desired in milk. Among the pathogens most commonly found in milk, the tubercle bacillus is the most heat-resistant. Therefore, a heat treatment that is sufficient to kill this organism is adequate to kill the other pathogenic organisms. A large amount of careful bacteriological investigation has shown that the tubercle bacillus will be killed when subjected to a temperature of 140° F. (60° C.) for 20 minutes. Today it is customary to pasteurize with a heat treatment of 142° F. (61.1° C.) for 30 minutes.

Now back to Cayce:

"(Q) Can Milk and Dairy Products be included in diet? Also eggs?

"(A) The yolk of eggs might be taken, but not so well for the whole egg. Milk products may be gradually added, but for the body yet it is much preferable to use Dry Milks or Malted Milks rather than Raw Milk."

We have already read how the whites of eggs produce an acidic condition in the body, which Cayce wanted to avoid, seeking to maintain a slightly alkaline condition. See the section on Acid and Alkaline Balance on pages 80-85.

"(Q) Is it well for the body to refrain from eating all dairy products, with the exception of butter and cream, and substitute a Soybean Milk for a beverage?

"(A) For this body in the present, it would be very well. Though the Soybean Milk product is not well for EVERY body, in these particular conditions here it is very good; especially owing to the reactions through the assimilated forces from same for the heart activity." (1206-8)

As we see in this Cayce reading, he is recommending an alternative to cow's milk. Today the alternatives to cow's milk are almond, soy, and rice milk. Each of these milks has its advantages and disadvantages. And that very much depends on a person's body – as Cayce noted in the reading, saying that for this body soy milk was okay but it was not for everybody.

Two other alternatives to cow's milk are found in his readings. One is a common alternative: goat's milk. But the other is a surprise: mare's milk!

—Goat's Milk and Mare's Milk—

"This should be goats' milk or mares' milk. If goats' milk or mares' milk may not be obtained, then use the DRY milk - rather than raw milk, or even that that has been pasteurized." (4320-3)

"(Q) Do you advise goat milk for the body?

"(A) It's very good. Mare's milk would be better, if you want the best for the body!" (631-7)

To my surprise mare's milk is available online – mostly for feeding rejected or orphan foal (a young horse). Most of it is sold as a freeze-dried powder. Mare's milk has long thought to have curative properties, touted as a balm for digestive problems, elixir for the liver, a tonic for general malaise and great for the skin. Human infants with severe food allergies will often tolerate mares' milk when all other milk makes them sick. Recent research suggests that this is because mares' milk is closer in composition to human mother's milk than that of any other mammal! (Issue 2608 of *New Scientist* magazine, 16 June 2007, page 58)

In central Asia, mare's milk is a staple food, though they prefer it with a kick. In Mongolia, Kazakhstan and Kyrgyzstan the tradition is to ferment it in a horse-hide sack for a few days until it turns into a frothy, acrid, and mildly alcoholic beverage called *kumis*, or *airag* in Mongolia. I'll leave this decision up to you.

Studies done at the USDA and Prairie View A&M University link goat's milk to an increased ability to metabolize iron and copper, especially amongst individuals with digestion and absorption limitations. Another main health benefit of goat milk is that it is closer to human milk than cow's milk making it easier to digest and assimilate in the human body. The size of the fat molecules in goat's milk are much smaller than those found in cow's milk, again making it easier to digest. Goat's milk also provides high amounts of calcium, the amino acid tryptophan, with fewer side effects than cow's milk.

Here is a brief pro and con for each of the common milks sold in our grocery stores:

—Cow's Milk—

Cow's milk remains one of America's most common daily drinks, but it may be one of the sources for gas, bloating, and other forms of indigestion. The average cow is given growth hormones, antibiotics, GMO feed, vaccinations, and exposed to toxic conditions.

Whole cow's milk with none of the fat removed contains 8 grams of fat per cup, 8.5 percent nonfat milk solids, and 88 percent water. As none of the milk's helpful components are removed through pasteurization, it is high in natural proteins, fat, calcium, and vitamin D, all of which are important.

Of course many dairy milks have some or all of the fat removed. There are 150 calories in one cup of whole milk. The 1 percent variety of milk has 110 calories. And "skim" milk has just 80 calories. Fat-free milk has all of the nutritional benefits of whole milk without the saturated fat and calories.

There is also Lactose-free milk for those people who cannot break down lactose, a natural sugar in milk products. As with the other dairy milks, lactose-free milk is a good source of protein, calcium, vitamins, and minerals.

The negative elements of milk are high in saturated fat and calories (if the fat is not removed), and high cholesterol.

—Almond Milk—

(Personal note: I do not like manufactures calling drink products "milk" when they do not come from a mammary gland! But alas it is a marketing game and there is little that can be done.)

Almond milk is made from ground almonds and is lower in calories than other milks as long as it is unsweetened. It's also free of cholesterol, saturated fat, and is naturally lactose free. Even though almonds are a good source of protein, almond milk is not. Almond milk is also not a good source of calcium. It takes about 2 cups of almonds to make a half gallon of almond milk; however, the grounded almonds are strained through water, so we aren't getting much of the almonds. Most of it is water.

Because of the way it is made it is not a good source of protein and, unless it is fortified, it contains no calcium, which is important for people with conditions like osteoporosis. Also people who are allergic to almonds or nuts should avoid almond milk.

—Soy Milk—

Here is a product this surrounded in controversy, with proponents and detractors. Yet, our stores are full of soy products. From my own research I have been unable to clearly determine who has the truth about soy – is it healthful or harmful. You must be your own judge on this.

Soy milk is a popular milk alternative for vegans and people who are lactose intolerant. Since it comes from soybean plants it is naturally free of cholesterol, low in saturated fat, and contains no lactose. Soybeans and soy milk are a good source of protein, calcium, and potassium.

However, too much soy can be a problem for those with thyroid disease and other conditions. A 2008 Harvard study showed that higher intakes of soy-based foods caused fertility problems and lower sperm counts. Thousands of studies link soy to malnutrition, digestive distress, immune system breakdown, thyroid dysfunction, cognitive decline, reproductive disorders and infertility, even cancer and heart disease. A primary reason is the high levels of phytic acid in soy, and this can reduce *assimilation* of calcium, magnesium, copper, iron, and zinc. Another reason is the fact that more than 90 percent of soybeans grown in the United States are genetically modified. Genetically modified foods (GM) were introduced in 1996. Some researchers are concerned that the increase in low birth weight babies, infertility, and other problems in the U.S. may be a result of these genetically engineered foods.

Also, *unfermented* soy has also been linked to gastric distress and chronic deficiencies in amino acid uptake, which can result in pancreatic impairment and cancer. Unfermented soy is also loaded with phytoestrogens, which can actually alter a woman's menstrual cycle. This compound mimics and sometimes blocks the hormone estrogen, and has been found to have adverse effects on various human tissues, particularly in women's bodies. (Some sources see Western women's bodies as being different than Asian women, and therefore soy's influence in their bodies is different.)

Opposing the detractors and negative reports there is another body of researchers claiming the healthy view: that soy products are good for women, even Western women.

As best that I have been able to determine, any soy that is not fermented is not a health food. I know some people will be upset with me but I have tried to be as objective as possible.

Traditional *fermentation* of soybeans destroys the anti-nutrients in soybeans. Even organically grown soybeans naturally contain phytic acid, which contains the anti-nutrients saponins, soyatoxin, phytates, trypsin inhibitors, goitrogens and phytoestrogens. Fermented soy products include: Nattō, Miso, Tempeh, Soy sauces, *fermented* tofu and *fermented* soy milk (most soy milk and tofu in the U.S. is *not* fermented).

Note: there is some confusion as to whether some store brand tofu is fermented or not. Unfortunately, tofu products vary greatly in their compositions because there is no established standard.

Miso is a fermented form of soybean and is rich in such soy nutrients as isoflavone aglycones, genistein, and daidzein, which are believed to be healthy. However, traditional miso starts with fermenting cooked *rice* with Koji spores (spores from *Aspergillus Oryzae*). Many believe that Mugi barley miso is better than the rice processed miso (I think Cayce would agree). Barley is better. However, Genmai miso uses whole-grain *brown* rice instead of white rice, and Cayce clearly would support this.

Nattō contains an enzyme produced in the fermentation process called *nattokinase*, which is a powerful agent contained in the sticky part of Nattō that dissolves blood clots that lead to heart attacks, strokes, and senility. Nattō also contains vitamin K2 and isophrabon, which help to prevent diseases such as osteoporosis and breast cancer and slow down the aging process. However, Natto's smell, flavor, and its slimy texture is challenging for some people to accept.

Tempeh's fermentation process and its retention of the *whole* bean give it a higher content of protein, dietary fiber, and vitamins – particularly B-vitamins. It has a firm texture and has an earthy flavor which becomes more pronounced as it ages. It is often in loaf form.

The fermentation process reduces the phytic acid in soy, which in turn allows the body to absorb the minerals that soy provides. (One source: Amanda Rose. "Soy and Phytic Acid: Stick with Fermented Tempeh and Miso".)

—Rice Milk—

Rice milk is made from milled rice and water. It is the least allergenic of all of these products. While rice milk can be fortified with calcium and vitamin D, it is not a natural source of either of these, just like soy and almond.

Unfortunately, rice milk is very high in carbohydrates and very low in protein, so it's the least desirable choice for people with diabetes as well as people who want more protein, such as athletes and the elderly.

—Butter Fat & Cheese—

"(Q) What causes nerve pain below shoulder blades on right side of spine?

"(A) This is a part of those disturbances from the digestive forces. A little fat, here, needs to be taken; especially as from butterfat or dairy products."

"(Q) Should she eat a butter made of vegetable oils or dairy butter?

"(A) Vegetable oils the better. Much nuts and nut fruits may be used also. All it (the body) will assimilate." (4281-14)

"It would be well, as we find, for the body to refrain from great quantities of butter fats or milk, or cheese, or any of those things that carry ... the activity of the liver in the emptying or pouring into the system fats of any kind that cause the rash, or the eczema that appears as a rash on parts of the body.

"(Q) Do olives affect body?

"(A) Depends upon their combinations. Olives with meats, as fowl or the like, are very good. Olives with potato salad or with those that have any great quantity of acid, are harmful. Helpful in other directions.

"(Q) How about cheese with olives?

"(A) Depends upon whether there's anything harmful in the cheese; whether it's the white cheese or whether the brown breads or whether those cheeses that are made from the perfectly soured milk or curds or whether they are those that carry some other properties." (257-170)

The same man later asks:

"(Q) What cheeses are best?

"(A) Those that are the more easily assimilated by the system; as all of the products of the better cheese processes; not too much of a Cheddar nature, or that is too soured." (257-225)

"DO be consistent with the diets – keeping away from pastries, cakes and the like, and too much starches - for instance, spaghetti and cheese; though cheese may be taken in moderation if it is a cream or cheddar cheese. DO NOT eat white potatoes. DO NOT eat white bread." (459-11)

"(Q) What about cheese?

"(A) Cheese is not as well for the body, this particular body, as some others; unless it is fresh - and this is not as palatable to the body as others. Yogurt and such combinations, which arise as the basis for cheese, is very good; especially for the colon condition. Honey in the honeycomb, and only with the comb, should be the greater part of that taken as sweets. A stimulation occasionally as of wine with bread, not as a drink but just as a potion to bring rest to the body. When taken it should only be taken with rye or sour or brown bread." (846-1)

"(Q) Is cheese alright in the diet?

"(A) Alright if it isn't over-indulged in, or whole meals made on same. It depends also upon the character of the cheese. Cream cheese, or that made at home is very well; provided it is not too strong." (2743-2)

"(Q) What cheese?

"(A) Cream, Old English - as a cream - the American cheeses; all are very good, NOT in excesses." (257-167)

In another of his dietary overviews he made this comment about our favorite macaroni and cheese (oh poo):

"In the diet keep away from too great quantities of starches. Never take white bread, macaroni and cheese or white potatoes, though the jackets of the white potatoes would be well for the body. Yams (sweet potatoes) would be very well for the body; but not the bulk of white potatoes, white bread nor macaroni with cheese. Not red meats of any kind. Plenty of fish, fowl and lamb may be taken and a great deal of raw vegetables. Do these and we will bring better conditions for the body." (3620-1)

—Sweets—

For Cayce sweets were a cause of acidity in the body's chemical soup. And when combined with starches, such as breads, pastries, and starchy vegetables, they negatively affect the body. He favored eating sweets with meats, and then in moderation. Here are some of his directions:

"In the diet, keep to more of an alkalin-reacting diet. Not great quantities ever of condiments, as highly seasoned foods, great amount of spices or a great amount of starch WITH pastries, pies or the like. Ice cream or ices may be taken. The sweets taken should be at the time meats are eaten, rather than at the time when breads are taken. Beware of potatoes in any form, unless they are roasted or baked with the jackets on and more of the jackets are eaten than of the core or the center of same." (1178-1)

As viruses enjoy an acid environment, he recommended the following to someone who already had the cold virus:

"As we find, there is rather an acute condition of cold or congestion from an unbalancing in the alkalinity of the system. Not by the foods themselves; rather the manner of their *combination*. For, as indicated, there should not be taken starches and sweets at the same meal, or so much together. That's why ice cream is so much better than pie, for a body!" (340-32)

Again we see his concern about food combinations rather than foods per se. Combining sweets with starches was not a healthy mixture.

"Not too much of the white breads, especially with sweets. Meats with sweets; only those meats, however, of fowl or lamb - occasionally fish." (1058-2)

In the following discourse we see him not wanting to totally eliminate sweets from a diet, preferring rather a moderate balance.

"(Q) Should I eliminate meat and sweets from my diet?

"(A) These may be curtailed, but to eliminate entirely as we find would create an unbalanced condition in the chemical reaction of the bodily forces. No FRIED meats; and honey should be used principally as the sweets. Fish, fowl or lamb would be the principal meats; and the fish fresh, and the lamb roasted, - all of these boiled, roasted, baked or broiled, but never fried." (1620-3)

Combination of foods was important but so was quantity, as in this directive:

"Do not eat great quantities of starch with the proteins or meats. If sweets and meats are taken at the same meal, these are preferable to starches." (416-9)

"Keep the eliminations near normal, with the diets towards a tendency of the alkalin-reacting rather than large quantities of meats or sweets - but these taken in their proper proportions. Eat the sweets rather with meats than with breads." (533-11)

Cayce was in favor of the sweetness found in fruits and vegetables: "The fruit sweets, or natural sweets, or vegetable sweets, are the better for the body." (632-7)

"Keep away from too much starch, too great a quantity of sweets; save natural sweets, as from fruits, vegetables, the small fruits such as berries and things of that nature, and honey." (543-24) —like turkey and cranberries, yum!

—Fats—

I know what you may be wondering: did Cayce suggest eating fats? Yes, in healthy cases he did; as does the American Heart Association: "Dietary fats are essential to give your body energy and to support cell growth. They also help protect your organs and help keep your body warm. Fats help your body absorb some nutrients and produce important hormones, too. Your body definitely needs fat." (April 28, 2016)

Cayce did see an important role for fats in our diets. Here are some of his comments:

"(Q) What is the cause and remedy for pain under right shoulder blade?

"(A) This comes from the lack of those proteins in the system to make the ducts properly vibrate in their respective forces. Hence some fats, as may be taken occasionally, will relieve these disorders. Fats as of beef fat, mutton fat, turkey fat, goose fat, hare fat, or the like." (543-15)

"With fats be sure that the sweets are taken at those periods also; or sweets such as honey, not sweets made with corn starch or cane sugars should be used.

"(Q) Do you mean that when fats are taken the sweets should be taken also?

"(A) Sweets such as honey, if or when fats are taken. The fats should be from fowl; not from swine nor kine [cows]." (974-1)

Eat "sufficient protein, fats, and vegetable forces to supply the needs of the carbon and the fats for the body." (538-12)

I must add here that many of Cayce's more severely ill questioners were told to avoid all fat because their digestive systems could not properly digest and assimilate it. In their case fats (and he often added "greases") would cause more problems than the lack of fat in their diet. He wanted them to first improve their digestive system, then add the protein and fat to the diet.

—Ingestion is one Thing
Assimilation is quite Another—

Keep in mind that ingesting a food does not automatically mean that our bodies received any benefit from it. What we ingest needs to be *assimilable*. Assimilation is the processes whereby our cells are truly supplied with the nutrients needed for life, vitality, and renewal.

There are 2 ways our bodies assimilate food value: (1) by absorbing vitamins, minerals, and other chemicals from food as it passes through our gastrointestinal tract (the esophagus, stomach, and our small and large intestines). Our bodies do this by causing a *chemical* breakdown using enzymes and acids, and a *physical* breakdown by oral mastication (chewing and mixing food with the enzyme amylase, also called ptyalin) followed by the muscle of the lower part of our stomach mixing the food and liquid with its digestive juices (enzymes pepsin and rennin, hydrochloric acid, and mucus). Then, our small intestines mix food with digestive juices from the pancreas, liver, and intestine (bile from the liver and from the pancreas a clear alkaline digestive fluid with a variety of enzymes, including trypsinogen, chymotrypsinogen, elastase, carboxy-peptidase, pancreatic lipase, nucleases and more amylase). The jejunum (between the duodenum and ileum) is the middle section of the small intestine that serves as the *primary site of nutrient absorption.*

Then the small intestines push the mixture forward to help with further digestion.

(2) The second process of bio assimilation is the chemical transformation of substances in our *bloodstream* using liver and cellular secretions. The assimilability of many compounds is dictated by this second process since both the liver and cellular secretions can be very specific in their metabolic action on a variety of foods.

We may think of these 2 processes as one being our gastrointestinal tract and the other being a process occurring in our blood and liver.

Keep assimilation in mind when choosing and eating foods. Consuming more easily assimilated nutrient-rich foods means we do not have to eat as much as when we eat processed, refined, empty-nutrient foods that are packed with sugars, additives, and preservatives. For example, we can stuff ourselves at a restaurant with white French bread before our entrée and fill full; but our body still wants to eat! Why? Because the white bread has little to no useful nutrients in it, so our body did not get what it needed. Even though we fill full *we are not nourished.*

Instead of eating the convenient, fast, refined foods available to us today we would be so much healthier if we were ingesting and assimilating raw, alkalizing foods that shift our diet to fresh fruits, vegetables, and whole grains. And here's a side benefit: we would weigh less! America has become overweight because of its reliance upon fast, convenient, processed foods. These are low in nutrients.

Many foods in our diets (mostly meats and starches) leave us feeling sluggish and needing to rest after eating. However, fruits and vegetables are mostly water, vitamins, minerals, water-based fats (such as in avocado) and fiber. Some have complex sugars, like apples. Admittedly we have found that diets rich in vegetables and fruits can challenge some bodies due to the high amount of fiber in these foods; so you have to discover how your body does with high-fiber foods. In most cases our bodies do adjust to eating fiber-rich diets.

Greens. either raw or cooked, contain fibers that are easily assimilated and more tolerable than some veggies like broccoli. Greens like kale, arugula, collards, chard, kale, romaine, are easily assimilated and provide nutrients. We don't need a lot of greens to get a lot of benefit. They provide high quality nutrients such as iron, vitamins A, C, and K, and even a little protein. Put them in a salad, steam them, make soups of them, and of course add them on the side with an entrée.

Green beans are more like a vegetable than a bean, and they are assimilable. Very low in carbs and free of starchy sugars, they're very simple to digest unlike pintos, kidneys, and black beans (which are still good but not as easily assimilated as green beans). Green beans are also packed with nutrition such as fiber (3 grams), protein (4 grams), and Vitamin C (20 percent) in just one cup.

Here's a little tidbit of info: Sugars inhibit the secretion of ptyalin, an enzyme in the saliva for the digestion of starches. When sugars and starches are combined, the starches cannot properly be digested because the sugars inhibit the production of the needed ptyalin to process the starches. Sugars and starches should be eaten separately.

When a protein and starch are eaten in the same meal, the starch soaks up the stomach's powerful digestive hydrochloric acid that is meant for digesting the protein. This inhibits the digestion of the protein. Starches and proteins should be eaten separately.

As Cayce taught, combinations of foods are an important factor in determining what is good for our bodies.

I cannot give you a list of sugars that can be eaten with starches because there isn't one. But here is a list of non-starchy vegetables that could be eaten with proteins and not inhibit digestion:

Arugula, Yellow summer squash, Cauliflower, Green beans, Scallion, Zucchini, Celery, Kale, Lettuce, Parsley, Turnip greens, Brussels sprouts, Sorrel, Asparagus, Collard greens, Mung bean sprouts, Spinach, Bamboo shoots, Cucumber, Mushrooms, Sweet pepper, Beet greens, Dandelion greens, Mustard greens, Sweet corn, Bok Choy, Eggplant, Okra, Swiss chard, Broccoli, Endive, Onion, Turnip, Broccoli, Escarole, Fennel, Radishes, Watercress, Cabbage, Rhubarb, Seaweed, Kohlrabi, Snap beans, Chicory, and so on.

—Take Time to Eat for Your Body's Sake—

You may think that our modern life is the busy life but Cayce was having this problem back in the 1920s through the 1940s. People eating on the run – thus the term "fast food." Here's one of his directives:

"Take time to eat! Don't eat on the run! Sit down and be quiet during those periods when the food is being taken! Rest at least five to ten minutes before the food is taken at EACH meal! Don't hurry in; or run in, grab, and be gone!" (259-7)

—Other Elements of Diet and Health—
—Water!—

Water intake was very important to Cayce.

"Q: How much water should the body drink daily?

"A: At least sixteen glasses full!" (263-1)

And another:

"Q: Should I drink plenty of water, and how many glasses each day?

"A: Drink plenty of water. This as we find is most helpful to the body. Six, eight, ten glasses a day." (1196-9)

And since Cayce is also recommending more fruits and vegetables in our diets consider this information from "Healthy Eating" by Mala Srivastava:

"Reaching for a watermelon or cucumber after finishing an intense workout may hydrate your body twice as effectively as a glass of water, claims a 2009 study by researchers at the University of Aberdeen Medical School [a public university in Aberdeen, Scotland, founded in 1495!]. This is so because water-rich fruits and vegetables also provide you with natural sugars, amino acids, mineral salts and vitamins that are lost in exercise. The study found that this combination helps hydrate you more effectively than water or sports drinks. Eating fruits and vegetables high in water content can replenish your body without all the artificial colors and flavors commonly found in sports drinks. The biggest advantage of consuming high water content foods is that they contain minimal calories and provide a feeling of fullness."
(Source: http://healthyeating.sfgate.com/list-fruits-vegetable-high-water-content-8958.html)

In no way does this reduce or eliminate the need for plenty of water – plenty of water is need!

Our body's weight is approximately 60 percent water. Our body needs water in all its cells, organs, and tissues to help regulate temperature and bodily functions. We lose water through breathing, sweating, and digestion. We hydrate our bodies by drinking water, fluids, and eating foods that contain water. Water does more than just quench our thirst and regulate our body's temperature; it also keeps the tissues in our bodies moist. Keeping our bodies hydrated helps it retain optimum levels of moisture in sensitive areas (e.g., eyes, nose, mouth), as well as in the blood, bones, and the brain. Water also helps protect our spinal cord and acts as a lubricant to our joints.

Of course, we also have to consider *excess* water retention in our bodies as well. One of the biggest challenges to effectively losing weight is reducing the amount of water that the body retains. Many foods and beverages can act as natural diuretics for reducing water retention. The natural diuretics foods include: celery, parsley, watercress, cucumber, carrots, avocado, pineapple, and spices like fennel, ginger, and turmeric, and teas like red clover and those containing burdock root. And yes, caffeine in coffee and most teas is a diuretic as well.

—Supplements—

Supplements were recommended. Vitamins and minerals, as well as many rather unique and often curious additions were suggested. But overall, Cayce sought to gain the body's needs through foods ingested rather than pills. However, because of environmental changes and reduced soil quality, it may not be as easy today to get all we need without supplements. Another good reason to grow at least some of your own food, making sure to keep your soil enriched.

—Coffee & Tea—

Here again we find Cayce's advice to be founded on moderation. Both coffee and tea were included as part of a healthy diet.

"(Q) Is coffee or tea good for this body?

"(A) Coffee is better than tea, though the body may prefer the tea. Coffee without milk and without sugar is preferable; but coffee without cream or milk IS a food value. There is very little food value in tea, though it is a stimulant. Coffee is preferable." (462-6)

In an apparent contradiction of what he just said, he tells another person that tea is better. This is a clear example of how Cayce was influenced by the person seeking his help and their specific body and mind.

"Not too much stimulation of coffee or tea, but tea would be preferable over coffee." (81-2)

Generally, he considered tea to be less desirable than coffee, as in this next reading:

"(Q) Is tea and coffee harmful to the body?

"(A) Tea is more harmful than coffee. Any nerve reaction is more susceptible to the character of tea that is usually found in this country [U.S.A.], though in some manners in which it is produced it would be well. Coffee, taken properly, is a food; that is, WITHOUT cream or milk." (303-2)

Cayce's statement about tea being more harmful, especially in the U.S. is because of the amount of tannin in black tea. Today we have many teas that do not have tannin. Tannin is a yellowish or brownish bitter-tasting organic substance present in some galls, barks, and other plant tissues, consisting of derivatives of gallic acid, used in leather production and ink manufacture. The tannins in tea are called thearubigins, a class of chemicals that includes theaflavins. These chemicals are formed in black tea when the antioxidants inherent in green tea become oxidized. The tannins in tea have a negative impact on health in that the tannins inhibit the body's iron absorption. However, green and white teas, and low-oxidation oolongs tend to contain little to no tannins, although they are rich in catechins, which are pseudotannins.

There is tannin in coffee but it is of a much lower degree than black tea.

However, in several cases Cayce instructed the removal of tannin, as in these two examples: "coffee without the tannin – as Kaffa Hag or the like." (340-24) "If coffee is used it should be that with the tannin removed, such as Kaffa Hag." (677-1) Cayce is referring to Kaffee Hag, Caffe Hag, and Café Hag. Caffe Hag is a worldwide brand of decaffeinated coffee that originated in Bremen in Germany in 1906. It took its name from the company title Kaffee Handels-Aktien-Gesellschaft – Kaffee HAG for short. General Foods acquired the original German company in 1979. The spelling of Café HAG was standardized in the 1990s. Both Café HAG and Sanka are now owned by Kraft Foods, which merged with General Foods in 1990. Here is the curious part of this: Café HAG is known as a *decaffeinated* coffee, not a tannin-free coffee. Sanka is French for "sans caféine", meaning *without* caffeine.

An interesting difference between tea and coffee is how their caffeine affects our bodies. When tea is made its caffeine combines with its tannins, which causes the caffeine in tea to be released more slowly than the caffeine in coffee, thus tea has a longer effect upon the body. Also, in coffee the caffeine affects the blood through the coronary system, which increases heart rate. The caffeine in tea affects the cardiovascular system and the central nervous system! As Cayce noted, tea is indeed a greater stimulant than coffee.

Here are some more of his comments:

"Coffee or tea may be taken in moderation, but coffee without milk or cream and tea preferably with lemon instead of cream, as a stimulant." (579-1)

"Coffee, tea or milk may be taken in moderation. Do not use creams or milk either in the tea OR coffee; but these are to be used (coffee and tea) merely as stimulants." (1121-1)

"(Q) Can coffee and tea be used by this body without harmful effects?

"(A) No one can use them without AFFECTING the body. As to whether they are harmful or not depends upon the extent to which they are used. Use one or the other; don't use them both. Tea is more harmful than coffee. Coffee is a food if it is taken without cream or sugar, and especially without cream; and if taken without the caffeine - as Kaffa Hag, or the like - it's really a food for the body." (816-5)

Now that I have given a clear view of Cayce's discomfort with tea in our diet, let me give you his favorite and often recommended tea (in 298 documents in his files!). Yellow Saffron tea is Cayce's favorite tea for a improving health. Second to Yellow Saffron tea (in 120 documents) is Mullein tea. He mentioned these two teas as being helpful to the kidneys, lymph, lacteals, and digestive system as a whole.

—Pepper and Salt—

One important instruction from Cayce was to not season while cooking but only after the food is cooked: "All seasoning should be done with butter and salt or paprika (or whatever may be used as the seasoning) AFTER the foods have been cooked! The cooking of condiments, even salt, DESTROYS much of the vitamins of foods." (906-1)

When it came to pepper Cayce always favored red pepper over black. He particularly favored Cayenne pepper. Here are some of his comments on pepper:

"Keep that of the stimulus that gives the strengthening forces to the body through that of cayenne." (3751-14)

"Season, with salt and cayenne, no black pepper." (2553-2)

"Season well, but not with black pepper, but with salt and cayenne." (3751-6)

"Not black peppers nor of highly seasoned with salt, see - leave out those properties, only that of Cayenne or red peppers." (4536-1)

I had a fascinating experience related to this black and red pepper issue. I was driving along an old country road when I stopped at a Mom-and-Pop restaurant. While eating I overhead a local country guy sharing this story with his other local patrons:

"My mom showed us kids the best way to know what foods are good for us. She once put a box of black pepper and a box of red pepper on the window sill of the kitchen. A week later she told us to open the boxes. In the black pepper box there was only black pepper. But the red pepper box was full of bugs! Mom then asked us kids which of these spices does Nature eat? Well I have used red pepper ever since Mom made that powerful point!"

Now when it comes to salt, Cayce was totally influenced by the condition of the person seeking his help. In some cases he strongly stated "little to no salt" in their foods, while in other cases he recommended lots of salt and pepper (always red, most often cayenne). In one reading he stated a dislike of *seasoned* salts – but remember that statement could have been solely influenced by the condition of the person he was speaking to and their bodily condition.

—Tobacco—

When it came to tobacco use Cayce was against the way tobacco was being made but was aware of some benefit in pure tobacco, as was originally used by Native Americans and others. Here's an example:

"(Q) Is tobacco good?

"(A) Tobacco in moderation, as all stimulants, is not so harmful. However, over acidity or over alkalinity causes same to become detrimental.

"(Q) What brands of tobacco are best?

"(A) Just tobacco, and no brand, is best! In its NATURAL state it is preferable to any of the combinations that are ordinarily put on the market in package tobacco!" (462-6)

—Wine and Spirits—

When it came to alcoholic drinks Cayce had this to say:

"(Q) Any kind of intoxicating drinks?

"(A) WINE is good for all, if taken alone or with black or brown bread. Not with meats so much as with just bread. This may be taken between meals, or as a meal; but not too much - and just once a day. Red wine only." (462-6)

"Beware of too much alcoholic stimulants at ANY time; though red wine may be taken with BROWN or BLACK bread in the late afternoon (or at cocktail time) - but JUST red wine!" (849-13)

"(Q) Should he abstain from Rye and Bourbon entirely?

"(A) Very occasionally they may be taken, but not too great quantities at any time." (257-167)

"(Q) Can I drink alcohol?

"(A) As indicated, it is WELL for the body - provided, when it is taken, there are those foods that it works with in the digestive system. See? (492-1)

Curiously, a few times he recommended mixing warmed Apple Brandy with an egg yoke, and then adding milk. And sipping this as an energy drink! "Using just sufficient of the whiskey to cook the yolk of an egg." (303-28, and other readings)

He did seem to have a taste for quality:

"(Q) Any specific kind of whiskey?

"(A) Use good whiskey - don't use just corn or that colored. Rye, of course, is the better for such conditions or for such purposes.

—Weight—

Many of us today have to watch our weight, and many, many businesses exist to help us do this. Here is one little reading with a Cayce comment:

"When the body feels WELL, whether it is underweight or overweight, this is the preferable way and manner to judge. The adding of weight is the adding of those things that make for the excess of reserve in fats, starches and sugars. These are harmful to the body. So under the present existent conditions, it is not harmful to the body to be underweight, just so the strength and vitality is maintained." (462-6)

I like his focus on how we *feel* rather than how we *look*. I have known some wonderful people who have lived good, long lives and been portly or skinny.

—Weight Loss Aid—

One of Cayce's simple weight loss suggestions was taking a few ounces of watered-down grape juice before meals and bedtime. Here are 3 of those readings:

"(Q) Since she takes on weight so easily, what foods would be best in her diet?

"(A) Drink grape juice. This will keep down the weight. Take two ounces of grape juice (such as Welch's) and one ounce of plain water, half an hour before each meal is taken and just before retiring of night." (2084-16)

"Keeping way from starches will keep down the weight. Also taking Grape Juice about thirty minutes before each meal and before retiring at night, - two ounce of grape juice with an ounce of plain water (not carbonated, not distilled, but plain tap water and preferably Welch's Grape Juice), - this will keep down the sugars and the fats for the body." (2546-2)

"To aid in normalizing the weight, - take grape juice - the unfermented, to be sure; preferably Welch's; taken consistently in this manner: Take two ounces of the grape juice stirred in one ounce of plain water (not carbonated water) four times each day; half an hour before each meal and about half an hour before retiring at night." (459-11)

Keep in mind that at the time Cayce gave these readings there were few to no organic grape juices on the market. And most were from concentrate, whereas today you can purchase whole, organic grape juice not from concentrate. You decide.

Warnings

Cayce did have some warnings and directives to avoid when planning our meals.

—Fried Foods—

He would occasionally warn against certain methods of preparation: "No fried foods at ANY time." (677-2)

I could never find any clarity about his position on pan fried foods versus deep fried, so you'll have be your own judge on this. There are 3 types of cooking in oil or fat that are *not* deep frying: 1. Searing, 2. Pan-frying, and 3. Sautéing. Searing is done to give a crisp crust but retain a tender inside. It is done in a hot pan with a small amount of oil or fat (usually olive oil), allowing each side to sizzle until a light brown crust forms. Then baked to cook through. Pan-frying is done in a medium-hot pan without baking; therefore the food needs to cook all the way through in the pan. This method relies more on "steam" to help cook the food. Sauté literally means "to jump." Sautéing is done in a hot pan with ample amounts of oil or fat (usually olive oil) that is hot but not smoking. Into this pan is added the food and it cooks fast, which causes the food to "jump" around from the heat – thus the name sautéing.

—Bad Combinations—

Here's another of his warning comments: "Not white bread and potatoes at the same meal. Not quantities of sweets *with* white bread. The meats and sweets should be preferably taken at the same meal. It isn't so much WHAT the body eats as it is the COMBINATIONS that are taken at times. Beware then of those things. (1151-2) Here's one more: "But do not make bad combinations; that is, fried meats with starches or potatoes. Leave off any fried foods altogether. Do not use white bread, rice, potatoes, spaghetti, macaroni or the like at the same meal - any two of them at the same meal." (1217-2)

It wasn't long ago when nutritious food was widely considered to only be protein, carbohydrates, and fats. In fact, minerals, vitamins, and enzymes were all but ignored! And fiber? Well food processing companies would actually remove and discard fiber, considering it to be too coarse for our intestines. It wasn't until recently that all these other food elements were recognized as being important to healthy eating. Enzymes are actively involved in metabolism (the chemical processes that occur within a living organism in order to maintain life). Recently researchers have come to know the various enzymes needed to properly prepare foods for ingestion, digestion, and assimilation. And mixing foods requiring very different enzymes causes us to lose some of the benefits of these foods during the process of digestion and assimilation. This is one of the reasons for Cayce's concerns about bad combinations. His simple tips: meats with sweets (and not too many sweets) and vegetables with starches (and not too many starches). Avoid the meat and starches combination, and avoid starches and sweets combination.

And as you know, this is very hard to do in our society. For more on combinations see Assimilation on page 107.

—Meats—

"No *red* meats; that is, rare meats. In meats preferably use fish, fowl or lamb, rather than other types. Have three vegetables grown above the ground to one under the ground. Have one meal each day, if possible, with ONLY RAW vegetables. Nuts are good, but do not combine same with meats. Let them take the place of same." (1151-2)

Now he wasn't absolutely strict on this red meat directive, and in some cases encouraged the eating of some red meat. He even developed an energizing juice for the body called "beef juice." Beef juice is not a broth but a juice extracted from the meat through heat. It is prepared as follows: Take about one pound of round steak preferably. Cut off the fat, leaving the muscle and pieces of tendon. Cut this then into half inch cubes, and put it into a glass jar without water in it. The jar should be covered but not tightly. Put a cloth on the bottom of the pan to prevent the jar from cracking. Then put the jar into the pan with water in it – the water coming about one-half or three-fourths of the way toward the top of the jar. Let the water then simmer for three to four hours. Then strain off the juice which has accumulated inside the jar and the remaining meat may be pressed somewhat to extract the remainder of the juice. The meat will then be worthless. The juice should be taken two to three times a day, but not more than a tablespoon at one time, and this should be sipped very slowly taking perhaps five or ten minutes to use the whole amount. It may be seasoned to suit the taste of the individual. It would be well also to use a whole wheat or rye cracker at the same time to make it more palatable. Place the juice in a refrigerator but never keep it longer than three days. The quantity made depends upon how much and how often the juice is taken. Cayce wants it taken like a medicine not a drink. (1343-2)

"Let the meats be rather fish, fowl or lamb. And the combinations of sweets - do not have too great a quantity of sweets with vegetables, but at times when meats are taken a little sweets may be taken." (1217-2)

"No hog meat that is flesh of any kind; no bacon that is not VERY crisp - and this only at the morning meal." (677-2)

"In the matter of the diet, keep away from too much greases or too much of any foods cooked in quantities of grease - whether it be the fat of hog, sheep, beef or fowl! But rather use the LEAN portions and those that will make for body-building forces throughout. Fish and fowl are the preferable meats. No raw meat, and very little ever of hog meat." (303-11)

—Spirituality Helps Physicality—

From Cayce's holistic viewpoint, improving the conditions of the body require physical activity, proper nutrition, a good mental attitude, and even some serious spirituality. Here's the ending of a dietary reading for a young lady: "To be sure it will require time, patience, persistence and consistency. It will also be necessary for the mental and spiritual attitudes to be in that way of never condemning self or others, but rather looking to that power which lies within to have every atom of the body and mind attuned to creative energies as in the Christ-Consciousness, of His abiding presence with you." (3694-1) Curiously, he told this same woman: "Do learn the promises of the Christ, the Savior; especially those given to man after He arose from the grave. For these are quite different from those given even in the hour before His trial and crucifixion." Now I looked into this a bit and found that Jesus did indeed give different advice after his resurrection than before. Specifically, he was much more focused on the power of the Holy Spirit, the "Spirit on High," the "Spirit of Truth," to give us what we really need. He felt this to such a degree that he basically told the disciples to wait for it. Do nothing. Just wait prayerfully to be imbued with the Spirit of God.

One other surprising thing that I noticed was, while in his resurrected body, Jesus actually asked his disciples and the holy women if they had any food for him to eat! And they did. They had fish and honey in the honey comb, which Jesus accepted and ate. This mild sweet and meat combo fits well with Cayce's diet, especially since the meat is among his top three (fish, fowl, or lamb).

Admittedly, we cannot know all the ramifications of Cayce's thousands of food comments, especially since he was so influenced by the conditions and circumstances of the persons seeking the readings. But we can get a fairly clear sense of what he felt was best for physical bodies living in various environments on this little blue planet of ours. I suggest that you take what you can, what fits for you and your situation. Spring and summer certainly provide us with the best opportunity to eat better and to eat foods grown in our local area.

—It is Worse to Worry about What We Eat—

One last little comment that is important to remember in these busy times: Cayce said that it is worse to worry about your eating than to eat wrong. Worry produces more problems than bad food. This does not negate everything we've learned about good food, but it clearly shows that the mind is the builder, the shaper of outcomes. Let's be mindful of our thoughts and attitudes. Cayce's holistic approach takes into consideration influences of the spirit and mind as we are feeding our bodies.

Chapter 7
Exercise and Rest

Fresh Air Walks

"[Be in the] air, sand, and water. These are needed more for the body than any other condition – sunshine and shadows. The body needs to get CLOSE to nature, with nature's curers – as will be found in sand, sunshine, water, woods. Such natures as this, and we will find, in three to four weeks, with such care of self, such taking of sunshine baths, of sand baths, of walks in wood, of communing with nature, and of introspection of self and duty to self and that owed to mankind and to God, through the efforts of the individuals themselves, there will be brought strength, power, force, vitality. Do that." 5618-5

"We must have more oxygen, so that the lungs will throw off the carbon from the body. He should be more outdoors, and take more bodily exercise; have more employment of the mind, to get it off of self, or to do something that will relax the body, not enough of course to wear it out – then the body will rebuild." (5707-1)

In the following we have Cayce's body exercise for improving the flow and coordination of circulation and nerve impulses:

"First we would begin with systematic activity or exercise for the upper portion of the body itself; that is, the head and neck exercise. Take this morning and evening for a minute or two minutes at each period; and we will find there will be a great change in the activities of the vision, the hearing, the throat. This would be the manner:

"Sit erect - of morning just before arising, and of evening just before retiring. Slowly, positively, bow the head (not the body) just as far forward as possible, three to four times. Then back just as far as possible, with the body being held erect. Then slow circular motion, two to three times to the right, three to fours time to the left. Then to the side, first the right and then the left. Then the circular motion again; slowly but consistently. This should be taken immediately on awaking in the morning, you see, before leaving the bed; and just before retiring at night - or when ready for bed.

"Also we would take specific exercise (this has nothing to do with the head and neck exercise; that is, it should be taken in addition to the head and neck exercise, see?), systematically, morning and evening; two to three minutes in the morning before dressing, and two to three minutes in the evening when prepared for bed - the stooping exercise; that

"Stand erect, gradually rise on toes, extending the hands above the head as the body takes the exercise; then gradually stooping. Not bending forward but stooping, holding the heels rather close together - stooping three to four times, holding the body erect. [He is using the term stooping to mean "inclining the body" rather than fully bending over.] Then the circular motion about the waist: Hands on the hip, bend the body forward, circle backward. All this for two to three to four to five minutes. [We call this exercise, "scrubbing the barrel." We imagine scrub brushes on our hips and that we are inside a barrel and as we rotate our hips we scrub the insides of the barrel. It is very good for the lower body circulation and stimulation, especially the lumbar section of our cerebrospinal column.]

"This exercise is much preferable to having adjustments mechanically made, until there is the strengthening of the muscular forces throughout this portion of the body.

"Be mindful of the diet, that there is kept not too much of acids - or acid-producing foods. Keep away from too many sweets. No combinations of fried foods or great quantities of red meat.

"Do these, and we will find we will in a few weeks bring a great deal of change.

"Then we would continue to keep these exercises systematically, in periods, of course, with occasionally a rest period from same; and we will bring better conditions for the system." (1497-4, 46 year-old man)

The following is one of Cayce's best and most frequently recommended exercises. I do this exercise often and it is so good for keeping the body limber. Cats are the greatest creatures for stretching! And this Cayce exercise is based on emulating cat-like stretches:

"No better exercises may be taken than the stretching exercise; as rising on toes - and this doesn't mean with shoes on! - on heels, rocking back and forth; stretching the arms upward, the bending exercises, what may be literally termed - and is termed by some - the cat-stretching exercises, which includes, of course, being able - (put very coarsely) - to do the split, be able to put the head on the feet, to put the feet behind the head, to make the head and neck exercises and all of those activities that may be said to be of the feline or cat exercise. To be sure, in the present period, present development, present conditions that exist, must be gone at gently; but be persistent morning and evening, working at it, still not letting it become rote, but purposeful." (681-2)

Here is how many of us do this exercise that he just alluded to: We stand up straight, we rock back-and-forth on the heels and balls of our feet ("balls" are the padded portion between the toes and the arch). Then we stand flat footed and begin to alternately reach for the sky with our arms and hands, stretching like a cat scratching on our carpet or on a scratching post. The stretch is so full that we roll up onto the balls of our feet with each alternating stretch. Next, we bend over and alternately stretch our hands to touch our toes, letting our knees bend and our butt move as we alternate from right foot to left foot. It does not matter if you cannot touch your toes, just *reach* for them and feel the stretch in your back.

Usually this stretching is followed by the "scrubbing of the barrel" exercise described above and the head-and-neck. These stretches are excellent for keeping the body limber and the circulating flowing.

Breathing exercises were also recommended by Cayce, even Yoga breathing. You can see in these next two readings how important it is to expel the contents of our lungs more fully and inhale fresh air. This is best done at an open window or outdoors.

Here is one of Cayce's breath exercise:

"As we find, the meeting not only of the physical forces but to produce and bring about the greater abilities in the mental attitude, would be through the breathing exercises; or the nature of STRETCHING exercise taken WITH the breathing that would make for keeping the body more near normal, increasing those necessary influences for the overcoming of the tendencies in the body for those disturbances as indicated. Such an exercise would be that described as the STRETCHING of the arms, the lower limbs, with the intake and the sudden exhale from the lungs themselves; that not only purifies the activity of the source of energizing – or the energies for the blood supply – but alleviates those tendencies for the pressures that are indicated in the cervical areas. We would keep this a little of morning and a little in the evening before retiring." (989-1)

Our lungs need to be supplied because they supply our blood:

"Enliven the supplying of carbon and of the oxidized oxygen or ozone to the blood supply as reached through the lung forces, see?" (4790-1)

"In the blood supply to the body we find this in the lungs proper does not receive the sufficient carbon to supply the system." (4550-1)

Here is one many of us could use help with:

"(Q) Any special exercises that can be taken to strengthen flabby abdominal muscles?

"(A) Walking, riding, swimming, AND massage." (480-2)

—Rest and Relaxation—

"More would the body find self able to rest were the body to learn or attempt to RELAX self two to three times each day." (1371-31)

"(Q) Does the body rest and relax as it should?

"(A) Keeps at a very high nerve tension. Necessarily, recently, has relaxed more than usual - yet the body while sitting or resting rarely relaxes thoroughly. This, of course, is necessary to the better condition of the body." (147-35)

"Play as well as work. Be able to relax. Change in the thought is as often as much rest physically as to rest from physical and still keep the taxation mentally. For the body suffers over-taxation - mental more often than physical, for from physical taxation, sleep will recuperate but a mental is akin to those of the spiritual that prevent the relaxation, save by change of thought which will bring a relaxation.

"(Q) What mental interests should the body have?

"(A) These have been given. The body should interest self in play of variety or nature that is appealing or interests self in things that are entirely different from the activities. It may be work but work-mental will make the mind grow if changed. For to become lopsided or in such a groove as that it worries to do. That which causes other thought. In the line of art. Any line of play. Any line of change of surroundings that does not tax the physical body to excess.

"(Q) What can my wife do to aid this condition?

"(A) Make suggestions, if he will only heed them." (257-62)

—Budgeting Time—

"If the body will budget its time more regularly, not as habit, but as regularity, we find it will give more time for ALL of those developments that are a part of the body's experience in the present. So much time for study, so much time for recreation, so much time for relaxation. And have the relaxation in the open when practical." (1206-14)

Budgeting our daily, weekly, and monthly time is one of the best ways to do *everything* well! Allotting time for work, play, rest, exercise, social interaction, as well as quiet reflection truly makes for a healthy, happy, and fulfilling life.

—Sleep—

When Cayce was asked about the importance of sleep he took off in a direction that no one expected. Here is that discourse (read slowly and pause occasionally to reflect):

"Now, with that as has just been given, that there is an active force *within each individual* that functions in the manner of a sense when the body-physical is in sleep, repose or rest, we would then outline as to what are the functions of this we have chosen to call a *sixth sense*.

"What relation does it bear with the normal physical recognized five senses of a physical-aware body? If these are active, what relation do they bear to this sixth sense?

"Many words have been used in attempting to describe what the spiritual entity of a body is, and what relations this spirit or soul bears with or to the active forces within a physical normal body. Some have chosen to call this the cosmic body, and the cosmic body as a sense in the universal consciousness, or that portion of same that is a part of, or that body with which the individual, or man, is clothed in his advent into the material plane.

"These are correct in many respects, yet by their very classification, or by calling them by names to designate their faculties or functions, have been limited in many respects.

"But what relation has this sixth sense (as has been termed in this presented) with this SOUL body, this cosmic consciousness? What relation has it with the faculties and functions of the normal physical mind? Which must be trained? The sixth sense? *or must the body be trained in its other functions to the dictates of the sixth sense?*

"In that as presented, we find this has been termed, that this ability or this function - that is so active when physical consciousness is laid aside - or, as has been termed by some poet, when the body rests in the arms of Morpheus - is nearer possibly to that as may be understandable by or to many; for, as given, this activity - as is seen - of a mind, or an attribute of the mind in physical activity - LEAVES a DEFINITE impression.

"The activity, or this sixth sense activity, is the activating power or force of the *other* self. What other self? That which has been builded by the entity or body, or soul, through its experiences as a whole in the material *and* cosmic world, see? or is as *a faculty of the soul-body* itself. Hence, does the subconscious make aware to this active force when the body is at rest some action on the part of self that is in disagreement with that which has been builded by that *other* self, then THIS is the warring of conditions or emotions within an individual. Hence we may find that an individual may from sorrow SLEEP and wake with a feeling of elation. What has taken place? We possibly may then understand what we are speaking of. There has been, and ever when the physical consciousness is at rest, the *other self* communes with the SOUL of the body, see? or it goes OUT into that realm of experience in the relationships of all experiences of that entity that may have been throughout the EONS of time, or in correlating WITH that as it, that entity, HAS accepted as its criterion or standard of judgments, or justice, within its sphere of activity."

Cayce is saying that when our outer self is in repose our other, inner, deeper, immortal self is free to communicate, and it communicates from place of timeless soul-life, bring all the experiences and perspectives of our more cosmic being. Because of this, sleep has the potential to be of profound importance to our present incarnate life.

"Hence through such an association in sleep there may have come that peace, that understanding, that is accorded by that which has been correlated through that passage of the selves of a body in sleep. Hence we find the more spiritual-minded individuals are the more easily pacified, at peace, harmony, in normal active state as well as in sleep. Why? They have set before themselves (Now we are speaking of one individual!) that that IS a criterion that may be wholly relied upon, for that from which an entity or soul sprang is its CONCEPT, its awareness of, the divine or creative forces within their experience. Hence they that have named the Name of the Son have put their trust in Him. He is their standard, their model, their hope, their activity. Hence we see how that the action through such sleep, or such quieting as to enter the silence. What do we mean by entering the silence? Entering the presence of that which IS the criterion of the selves of an entity!"

Here Cayce is making us aware of power of living according to an ideal, a standard that is more than physical, as is seen in our becoming aware that we (deep inside) children (sons and daughters) of the Creative Force or God of the entire universe. We are celestial beings incarnating temporarily as terrestrial, physical beings. With this as our criterion or measuring gauge, our touchstone, our standard, then the immortal inner self becomes more present in this life and we develop our so-called "sixth sense" that can better guide us and convey intuitive insights for health.

"On the other hand oft we find one may retire with a feeling of elation, or peace, and awaken with a feeling of depression, of aloofness, of being alone, of being without hope, or of fear entering, and the BODY-PHYSICAL awakes with that depression that manifests itself as of low spirits, as is termed, or of coldness, gooseflesh over the body, in expressions of the forces. What has taken place? A comparison in that 'arms of Morpheus,' in that silence, in that relationship of the physical self being unawares of those comparisons between the soul and its experiences of that period with the experiences of itself throughout the ages."

Cayce is saying that when the *outer* self goes to sleep feeling happy but wakes feeling oddly uncomfortable, then the *inner* self is not content with what is going on in the outer life.

"Hence we find oft individual circumstances of where a spiritual-minded individual in the material plane is suffering oft under pain, sickness, sorrow, and the like – the soul is meeting that which it has merited, for the clarification for the associations of itself with that whatever has been set as its ideal. If one has set self in array against that of love as manifested by the Creator, in its activity brought into material plane, then there MUST be a continual, continual WARRING of those elements. So, my son, let your lights be in Him, for these are the MANNERS through which all may come to an understanding of the activities; for, as was given, 'I was in the Spirit on the Lord's day. I was caught up to the seventh heaven. Whether I was in the body or out of the body I cannot tell.' What was taking place? The subjugation of the physical attributes in accord with its infinite force as set as its ideal brought to that soul, 'Well done, you good and faithful servant, enter into the joys of thy Lord. He that would be the greatest among you would be the SERVANT of all.'

"What, then, has this to do - you ask - with the subject of sleep? Sleep - that period when the soul takes stock of that it has acted upon during one rest period to another, making or drawing - as it were - the comparisons that make for Life itself in its ESSENCE, as for harmony, peace, joy, love, long-suffering, patience, brotherly love, kindness - these are the fruits of the Spirit. Hate, harsh words, unkind thoughts, oppressions and the like, these are the fruits of the evil forces, and the soul either abhors that it has passed or enters into the joy of its Lord. This an ESSENCE of that which is *intuitive* in the active forces. Why should this be so? How received woman her awareness? [he is referring to Eve in Genesis] Through the sleep of the man! Hence INTUITION is an attribute endowed WITH all of those abilities and forces of its Maker. In sleep all things become possible, as one finds self flying through space, lifting, or being chased, or what not, by those very things that make for a comparison of that which has been builded by the very soul of the body itself." (5754-2)

Whew! Where did that come from! It is clear that Cayce's mind saw us as much more than we realize and with great potential to fully become aware of the Creative Forces, the Forces of Cosmic Life flowing through us and enlightening us.

Let's end with this in one sentence of his:

"Sleep is the building time of the physical forces to give and partake of rejuvenal expressions." (5681-1)

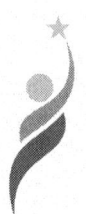

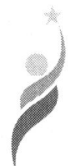

Chapter 8
Therapies, Tonics, and Devices

There is so much information in the volumes of Edgar Cayce's discourses on therapies, tonics, packs, and devices that it would take more than this book can convey. You will find most all of his information and much more on the EdgarCayce.org website, especially the section containing the Edgar Cayce Health Database. I encourage you to go to that website and search for what you need or want. Here I will highlight some of his main modalities for developing and maintaining health.

Massage

It may sound strange but from Edgar Cayce's perspective massaging the body can help spiritual enlightenment and attunement as well as physical health. And spirituality in turns helps develop and maintain health and wellbeing. Cayce tells one person that "the spiritual forces may be stimulated by massage, supplying energies from the various centers in the cerebrospinal system. This may be accomplished by massage." (3305-1) Cayce explains that "replenishing and rebuilding the ability to be in at-onement with the Creative Forces, or God, brings the ability to heal one's own self." (1861-15) Toward this end, he says that massage acts as an "assistant or booster to better attunement between the cerebrospinal and sympathetic nervous system." (1861-15) He identifies the cerebrospinal system with the kundalini pathway (sushumna) of ancient yoga meditation. He identifies the autonomic system with the seven chakras in the Yoga Sutras, and directly connects them to the seven endocrine glands that secrete the all-important hormones in our body. In reading 3098-1 he says that "massage will keep the centers and ganglia along the spinal system in better coordination." And in reading 2642-3 he says that "adjustments and massage will aid the body in its mental and spiritual attitude."

There are many types of massage, such as Swedish, neuropathic, osteopathic, lymphatic, and the Reilly method, which is taught at the Cayce-Reilly massage school and provided by trained therapists in the Cayce Spa at the center in Virginia Beach, Virginia, and of course all the graduates living across the country and practicing this method in your area. You can contact the Cayce Center to see if there is a Cayce-Reilly trained therapist near you. See illustrations on pages 211 through 223.

Generally speaking, Cayce is looking for a stimulating and coordinating massage throughout the body. This type of massage will improve balance and coordination. Remember, he is the father of holistic health and is always seeking that we have cooperation and coordination among our body, mind, and spirit. This for him was true health.

Here's an example from his files: "We find there are disturbances that prevent the body from its better physical functioning. These have to do primarily with that coordination between the sympathetic nerve system and the cerebrospinal nerve system." (3056-1)

The two important parts of our body to coordinate are the cerebrospinal, which is the kundalini pathway in yoga and the autonomic (sympathetic and parasympathetic) nervous system that includes the endocrine glands, and these are the spiritual centers or chakras in yoga.

The kundalini pathway is the area along the spine, from the base of the brain to the tip of the tail bone, and the extending nerves that exit out of the openings in the spinal column and to deliver and receive messages in a coordinated body. (illustrations: pages 211-223) Of course, it also includes the brain, especially the twelve paired cranial nerves.

The spiritual centers or chakras are located deep in the body and are part of the autonomic nervous system. These centers/chakras are stimulated and coordinated by *reflective* reaction to circular massage along the spine at the major plexuses. A nerve plexus is a branching network of intersecting nerves. They are located along our spine. A nerve plexus is composed of afferent (conducting toward) and efferent (conducting away) fibers that arise from the merging of the anterior rami of spinal nerves and blood vessels.

The root chakra and navel chakra are reflectively stimulated by circular massage throughout the lower back; the solar plexus chakra is stimulated by massaging the center of the back, the heart chakra by massaging between the shoulder blades, the throat chakra by massaging the neck. The higher two chakras located in the brain are stimulated and coordinated by massaging from the top of the spine, the base of the skull, over to the crown of the head (where our soft spots were when we first entered these bodies at birth), and then on to the forehead, the third-eye area. This is often referred to as Cranial Sacral Therapy, and is a gentle, noninvasive form of bodywork that addresses the bones of the head, spinal column, and sacrum. The goal is to release compression in those areas which alleviates stress, pain, and improves the flow of fluids and nerve impulses.

During the massage, it is important to keep one's consciousness near the Creator's, as indicated in this Cayce instruction: "General massage along the whole of the spine ... and keep that attitude that the applications are creating the field of activity in which the God-force or life itself may manifest in this body, that it may complete in this experience that development necessary for the maintaining of the soul's attitude and soul's relationships with its Creator and Savior." (632-2)

He wants us to use the massage time as a period of meditation, a period of attunement to the Divine within. Therefore, while the body is being enlivened and coordinated by the massage, direct the inner self to unite with the spiritual influences within. This will result in the best for body, mind, and spirit. In several discourses Cayce recommended that loved ones do the massage just before sleep. He explained that during the sleep cycle the body would be better able to rejuvenate itself, and the soul would be better able to reach higher dimensions of consciousness. On the following morning, do not move the body upon waking; rather, scan your deeper mind for a dream or, per chance, a vision.

Here is another of his readings for a person in which massage and spinal adjustments were encouraged:

"There has been, and exists in the present, incoordination between the nerve systems of the body. An over-anxiety, a fear has caused over-tension in the nervous system, especially as related to the areas in the upper dorsal [thoracic] or through the brachial centers, and has caused a great shock to the body, so that the ability of the nerves to coordinate in replenishing energies through the circulation has caused this great weakness which exists in the body." (5240-1)

It is important to note here that it was her emotions and mental state that affected her body. Therefore he also told her: "These may be materially aided but it will require as much activity of the mental self." She was going to have to get mental thoughts right if the physical adjustments were going affect a change in her health. See the mind-body connection here. This is often the case for us in healing and health, we need to improve our thoughts and emotions if our bodies are going to be truly healthy.

—Cayce's Therapeutic Oils—

Among Cayce's therapies are oils, most notably three: Peanut oil, Castor oil, and Olive oil. These oils were used to penetrate the body with their beneficial ingredients. The primary use of peanut oil in the Cayce readings was as a massage oil. It was described as a "food for the nerves and muscular forces" (2321-2) and a specific aid to joints. When Sassafras oil was added to it, it was an aid against arthritis. Castor oil was primarily used in a pack on the abdomen with heat, penetrating into the area of the major organs, most particularly the liver. In some cases the focus was on penetrating the intestines and the transverse colon. Olive was a food for the skin and body. Cayce noted that too much of olive oil would add weight to the body. All oils penetrate better with heat. In some cases a hot-water heating pad was used or an electric heating pad. But heat can also occur from the friction of massage, helping the peanut oil to penetrate. One of the problems with this therapy is the messiness of oils and how much oil Cayce wanted applied to the body. It is therefore best to set aside plenty of time for these therapies and select clothes that you don't mind getting oil on. Have a towel ready to rub off the excess oil once the therapy is completed.

Here are some of Cayce's comments about using these oils:

"(Q) Is peanut Oil best rubbing oil?

"(A) It is the best rubbing oil if sufficient of it is given for the body to absorb, for it becomes rancid less often than others." (257-233)

"(Q) Shall I resume peanut oil rubs?

"(A) There is nothing better. These may be given by any good masseuse. If they are taken once a week, it is not too often. For, they do supply energies to the body." (1158-31)

"Then have the rubdown with Peanut Oil, if the body would never have arthritis or neuritic reactions." (826-14)

"Those who would take a peanut oil rub each week need never fear arthritis." (1158-2)

"Massage with anything that is easy to massage with. If it is practical to obtain it, use Peanut Oil combined with an equal quantity of Olive Oil. Or, if Peanut Oil is not convenient, use an equal combination of Olive Oil and tincture of Myrrh; heating the oil to add the myrrh." (852-18)

"The activity of the olive oil [as a massage oil] is as FOOD that may be absorbed by the lymph and emunctories [an organ or duct that removes or carries waste from the body] of the system, provided the pores and the exterior portions of the body have been relaxed or opened before this is massaged into the system. The activity of those properties as go WITH same, the myrrh and those of sassafras oil, these add to the STRENGTH of the muscular tissue, of the sinew along the system, as to carry – the one stimulating the muscular forces, the other carrying to the cartilaginous forces, and to every nerve fiber itself, that of strength and activity." The Gold in its activity, with the Soda, is to ENLIVEN the glands INTERNALLY with the SECRETIONS of the system, as to furnish the proper stimuli to the replenishing and rebuilding of the system.

"We would massage along the cerebrospinal system equal parts of olive oil and tincture of myrrh, heating the oil to add the myrrh. Massage all that the cerebrospinal system will absorb." (372-8)

His Famous Castor Oil Pack

"We would apply hot Castor Oil Packs directly to the body, over the lower portion of the liver, the lacteal duct center, and extending to the caecum area. Use at least three thicknesses of flannel that is soaked or saturated in Castor Oil. Apply this as warm as may be handled comfortably, though not too hot. Then cover it with cloths, and an electric pad put over same." (2153-1)

"We would have the Castor Oil Packs over the lower portion of the liver, the gall duct, the lacteal duct, and extending to the caecum area. In these Castor Oil Packs we would use three to four thicknesses of flannel, as hot as the body can stand. These would be taken two or three days apart, for an hour at the time." (1055-1)

A pack was castor oil soaked into wool flannel.

Here is how I do my castor oil packs: I take a bowel into my bathroom and mix up the rising solution that Cayce recommended, which is some baking soda in warm water. I set a wash rag next to this bowel. Now I return to my bed. I turn on my large heating pad and place it on the bed in arms reach so I can get it once I have the pack on me. Then I prepare the bed with a thick towel covering the sheets so as not to soil the bed with oil. This first towel is right next to the side of the bed so I can get on it easily. Next to this towel I put a second towel in the middle of the bed. Then I prepare my pack on the first towel by laying out three side-by-side *overlapping* sections of plastic wrap from the kitchen so as to make a larger plastic section than the single sheets that come out of plastic wrap carton. This is my protective barrier for keeping the oil from getting all over the place. On this large plastic wrap I lay my large section of flannel folded three times for thickness. Then on this flannel I pour castor oil – wait until that soaks in – then pour on some more, making sure not to over soak the flannel so that it runs off and onto the towel and bed. Once the flannel has absorbed as much oil as it can hold, I lift it by the plastic wrap off of the first towel and put it to the side on the second towel while I get in the bed on the first towel (naked or with only underpants on). Then I carefully lift the plastic wrap and flannel and put it over my abdomen (the whole area as Cayce described it) flannel side on me. Then I lift up my heating pad and put it on the plastic wrap. Soon the pack gets hot. I lie back and am meditative and prayerful for an hour.

Now when I am done, I carefully removed the heating pad and turn it off. I carefully lift the pack off and set it plastic side down on the second towel. I go to the bathroom and wash the excess oil off of me using the rinsing solution and wash rag. Voilà! It is done. Now since the oil will not go rancid too quickly, I fold the pack into itself with the plastic wrap out and the flannel in, and put it in a plastic zip lock bag for future use. However, Castor oil is well-known to go rancid very easily and there is no way of telling because unlike other oils it does not give off a bad smell when it is rancid. I know people who keep using the same castor oil pack for many months but you may not want to reuse this pack for more than a month or two to insure that your oil is good. And each time you do reuse it, add fresh oil.

More information on castor oil packs can be found on the EdgarCayce.org website.

Hydrotherapy

Hydrotherapy is just what its name indicates: the therapeutic use of water. Cayce recommends several hydrotherapies, among them are Epsom salt baths, Sitz baths, steam baths, hot and cold showers, cabinet sweats, fume and vapor baths, enemas, and, yes, even colonics. The principal reason for hydrotherapy is to stimulate both blood and lymph circulation, coordination of our two main nervous systems, and to improve elimination of waste and toxins that develop in the body.

Anytime you are going to use hot water or steam, you should have someone close by to help you if your body reacts to the heat. And if you have any type of heart condition you should first consult your physician before beginning any hot water or steam therapies.

—Epsom Salt Baths—

Epsom salts baths were often recommended for persons suffering from muscular and joint pain or more serious conditions such as rheumatism and arthritis. Simply make a hot bath with plenty of Epsom salts dissolved in the water. Soak in this solution – it is very relaxing. Epsom salts are available at any pharmacy and some grocery stores.

—Hand and Foot Baths—

In most cases Epsom salts were used for hand and foot baths for symptomatic relief of arthritic or stress pain. Soak the hands or feet for five minutes, then massage them in the solution and work the fingers or toes, rotating the joints. Then soak again. Repeat for roughly twenty minutes.

—Sitz Bath—

A Sitz bath is for the hips and buttocks, the tail bone, pelvis, and hip joints, as well as the tissues in these areas of the body. Sitz baths are used for relief of pain, soreness, and discomfort in the pelvic and hip regions. There are three kinds of Sitz baths: a cold one, a hot one, and one that combines sitting in hot water first and then in cold water. Cold water should be between 60 and 65 degrees and the hot water between 100 and 105 degrees. The alternating of hot-and-cold baths should be done about three times in one session.

—Steam Baths—

Steam baths are use to sweat out toxins through our skin and lungs. Usually a steam cabinet or steam room is used at a spa. At Cayce's spa in Virginia Beach, Virginia steam cabinets are used. Various substances may be added to provide a vapor/fume that is absorbed through the opened pores in the skin. After the steam bath one would take a cleansing shower to rinse off the sweat and toxins on the skin.

Therapists trained in the Cayce/Reilly approach to giving steam baths are knowledgeable of safeguards and contra-indications for this form of hydrotherapy. It is usually best to begin with little heat to make sure that your body can handle the treatment. Gradually, greater heat can be used as the body indicates its ability to accommodate the heat and sweat.

—Hot and Cold Showers—

Here is a therapy that you can do right in your own living space for free: hot and cold showers. Our body's circulation of fluids and nerve impulses can be given a tremendous boost by alternating the flow of water from hot to cold, back and forth, over our bodies. The result is invigorating and healthful. Improving our circulation helps to relieve pain and feel more energetic. The hot water has relaxing properties, helping to reduce stress. Cold water helps relieve inflammation and stimulates the removal of toxins through elimination organs like the skin. When the body is subjected to cold external temperatures, the flow of circulation is directed *inward* toward the internal organs. As the outside temperature gets hot the flow of circulation goes *outward* toward the skin. Alternating hot and cold makes the circulation move in and out which releases stuck or sluggish fluid and stimulates nerve impulses.

Here are a few of Cayce's comments:

"When ready to retire, give first the shower of hot and cold water - one then the other several times - to get this shock that comes from such sudden changes to the exterior of the body." (1842-2)

"Do have the hot and cold shower. Do have the sitz baths. Do have a thorough massage with an equal combination of Olive Oil and Peanut Oil." (2621-3)

Here is advice to a young man needing more vigor but having a sensitive body: "Do not overheat the body nor make too quick changes through the cold showers, though hot and cold hydrotherapy would be well - provided it is supplied with plenty of massage during the application." (1123-3) While taking his hot and cold showers he should rub his body all over, enhancing the effects of the circulatory stimulation.

Hot and cold showers are an easy way to improve our circulation. Cayce occasionally recommended following these showers with a coarse towel rubbing up and down the spine on the back.

—Colonics—

I know how we do not like cleansing our colons with water and healthful substances, but Cayce recommended these.

"And keeping the colon clean is that which is necessary for every well-balanced body; hence should be a part of the experience for each entity." (1703-2)

Let me share my story with you.

Six years ago I had my first colonoscopy and they found 3 precancerous polyps and removed them. Three years ago I had my second colonoscopy and they found 4 precancerous polyps! I was heading in the wrong direction! So the colon therapists at the Cayce spa and I began a mild colonic schedule: one colonic each year with a GlycoThymoline (more on this Cayce product later) rinse at the end of each colonic. This year I had my third colonoscopy, and to my doctor's surprise and my joy there were NO precancerous polyps! The doctor asked what I had been doing, I told him, and he didn't say a thing, other than, "You don't need to come back for 5 years, and it would have been 10 years if you hadn't had 4 polyps just three years ago."

The only reason I had my first colonoscopy was because my friend and fellow staff member died of colon cancer, a cancer that could have been dealt with if only it had been found sooner. My friend was a healthy, energetic man - yet his colon took him down fast. Believe me when I tell you that when those precancerous polyps were found in my colon, and even after removing them they came back in greater number, I was scared and felt as though there was nothing I could do about it. Then when Dr. Oz announced on TV that he had 5 precancerous polyps on his first colonoscopy, and to his dismay and alarm about this - especially since he was eating and exercising and in good health. I was determined to try something beyond diet and exercise. I do not like colonics (who does) but I had no choice. Today, colonics with a Glyco-Thymoline rinse have become a part of my health regiment! By the way, both of my then-living parents (95 and 96 years old) never had any polyps, which actually caused me to be more alarmed at my situation.

While you lie on a cushioned table warm, filtered water is infused into your rectum and up your descending colon, flushed and then infused again, gradually reaching the transverse colon, flushed then infused again, gradually reaching the ascending colon. (illustration on page 223) The warm water circulates throughout the colon, dissolving and removing its contents, including particles stuck along the walls of the colon. Water temperature and pressure is closely monitored and regulated during a series of fills and flushes to generate the peristaltic action of the colon. A hospital gown ensures complete coverage for modesty and warmth. As the method involves an enclosed system, the waste materials are removed without the unpleasant odors or discomfort usually associated with enemas. A final rinse with Glyco-Thymoline promotes an alkaline environment in your colon. And as we have already read Cayce states that cancer cannot live or grow in an alkaline environment.

GlycoThymoline has been around for over 100 years. It was in 1890 that pharmacists Samuel Owen & Oscar Kress develop GlycoThymoline. It is a natural, healthful alkaline cleansing solution containing water, glycerin, alcohol (only 3.27%), sodium borate, sodium benzoate, sodium bicarbonate, carmine, sodium salicylate, menthol, eucalyptol, Abies Sibirica (Fir needle) oil, thymol, and methyl salicylate. As you can see the key ingredients are glycerin, menthol, eucalyptol, Fir needle oil, and thymol. Cayce recommended it many times for its alkaline properties.

A colonic should only be given by trained professional. Enemas are not as thorough as colonics but if colon therapy services are not available, then they will due. And local pharmacies have these available with instructions for self-application.

Tonics

Cayce designed some interesting tonics, potions, elixirs, and concoctions for improving health. Here are the main ones:

—Cayce's Spring Tonic 545—

He said "this would be good for everyone as a spring tonic." It is sold using various names. The official Cayce supplier calls it New Seasons Tonic. This herbal tonic is blended to aid digestion and assist in clarifying the whole system, especially during seasonal changes. It is an herbal tonic containing: Tolu Balsam Tincture, Wild Cherry Bark, Sarsaparilla Root, Yellow Dock Root, Dogwood Bark, Prickly Ash Bark, Dog Fennel, Sassafras Oil, Tincture of Capsici (Capsicum), Water, Grain Alcohol (7%).

Cayce first gave this formula to a nineteen-year-old female (Ms. 5450) to help her improve her body's overall chemistry and lower her toxicity levels. Initially it was called Tonic 5450, and is considered to be a good tonic for everyone.

—Cayce's Energy Tonic 636—

Tonic #636 is an herbal *energy* tonic for revitalizing and as a "beautifier," says Cayce. Its formulation is designed to support healthy digestion, particularly healthy *glandular* function (as in the endocrine glands we wrote about earlier). It contains a simple syrup (sugar) base blended with Elixir of Lactated Pepsin, Liquid Liver Extract, Fluid Extracts of Black Snake Root and Wild American Ginseng, Atomic Iodine, and Grain Alcohol (7-15%). It is very important to note that each 1/2 teaspoon provides .225mg or 150% of the Recommended Daily Allowance of Iodine! Iodine overdose is dangerous, so seek the advice of a health care professional before taking iodine supplements and do NOT use an iodine supplement or a supplement containing iodine in conjunction this tonic. Look at what your are ingesting in your supplements before taking this tonic. If a skin rash develops discontinue use and consult a physician (some people may be sensitive to iodine). If you are pregnant, nursing, have high blood pressure or a thyroid condition, seek the advice of a health professional before using this product. Dosages greater than 1/2 teaspoonful daily will supply iodine in excess of the Recommended Daily Allowance. Now with all of that said, this can be a very helpful tonic when taken properly.

Devices

Cayce designed and/or recommended several devices for aiding physical health. I am only going to give two of them here. You can find more on the EdgarCayce.org website.

—The Electric Massage Vibrator—

There are so many Cayce readings suggesting the use of a massage vibrator that it is among his most recommended devices. Here are some of his comments:

"These may be best balanced by a massage that would equalize the centers as indicated; in the 4th and 3rd dorsal area, 4th, 3rd and 2nd cervical area, and in the lumbar area. These centers may be stimulated sufficiently by the use of the electrically driven vibrator, provided there is sufficient heat applied before the application to draw circulation to those particular centers - see? Though the application would be, of course, along the whole cerebrospinal system, particular attention should be given in the particular centers mentioned, with the heat - preferably wet heat - applied first; and the application would be made about three times each week." (375-1)

In this next reading you will see him mention the Violet Ray device. More on this in a moment but notice his use of an electric massager.

"At times we would continue to use the Violet Ray, as well as the vibratory forces of the electrically driven vibrator. Do not use these in such a manner as to JUST get through with taking the treatment, but use them in such a manner as to accomplish a definite purpose at the time of the application of same. Take the electrically driven vibrator when tired, or before retiring; but don't wait too long to retire until it is too late to give the vibrator treatment!" (303-11)

This the reading that I follow closely, having my long-handled massager next to my bed to use up and down my spine just before sleep:

"In the evenings also before retiring, the use of the electrically driven vibrator along the whole cerebrospinal system will be found to be helpful; for this will enable all centers along the cerebrospinal system to receive a greater impulse from their activity, enabling all organs to be stimulated without the excess of one's functioning so much under the strain of the tautness of another. Especially would this be helpful, that those centers in the upper dorsal and cervical area receive stimulation; also across the lower portion of the body, or the lumbar area." (265-6)

These days it is difficult to find a long-handled massage vibrator. The people at Baar Products carry one, stock number 4290 (Baar.com).

"We would find that the electrically driven vibrator would be excellent for quieting the nerve forces of the body, ESPECIALLY in those areas over the plexuses indicated; that is, the upper dorsal and whole of the cervical area, and over the lumbar and sacral area." (369-10)

"Every day, preferably in the evening, use the Electrically Driven Vibrator across the lower portion of the cerebrospinal system, from the base of the brain to the end of the spine. Use the applicator that forms a suction upon the body itself; that is, the cup applicator. Then, use it across the abdomen; following the line of the colon, from the liver area down to the caecum, or opposite the right hip bone, then up and across the abdomen just below the navel and then down to the left side opposite the left hip bone. If these instructions are followed, it will require about fifteen to eighteen to twenty minutes. Don't just run the vibrator over those areas, but take time to give a thorough treatment. Come down, you see, along the cerebrospinal system - that's along the backbone, on either side of the backbone, and especially across the lower portion of the PELVIS area - that's across the small of the back and to the end of the spine! COME DOWN the spine, you see, with the strokes; not just running the machine back and forth! Then use it across the ABDOMEN, coming down from the liver area on the right side to the caecum, or that area just below or opposite the right hip bone. Then up just a little farther, you see, to the left; to that area directly below the navel area but on the right side. Then cross under the navel to the left portion of the colon. This is following, of course, the course of the colon." (1572-1)

Now this following reading reveals how our spirit/soul forces can influence our body's condition, and Cayce gives an interesting recovery process using the vibrator.

"This causing at this time a suppression of the action of the nerve forces to the cerebrospinal and produces despondency, but it is not an action of the brain itself, but it is a reflex sympathetic reaching through the soul and spirit forces, rather than to the building of the body itself. These are the conditions as we find them in this body here. Now, to give the proper balance to this body, and to relieve the conditions in this system, we would give it a systematic treatment along the sacrum and lumbar region, and to that of the whole length of the spinal column to some extent, and deep vibrations should be given from an electrically driven vibrator to this portion of the body to relax, and to the sacrum and lumbar and solar plexus and 9th dorsal deep vibrations; either side of the spine itself, and down to the knees, and that is the inside of the body lying on the face when this treatment would be given, and to the knees themselves and along the whole length of the sciatic nerve, and this will give the vibration to all of the organs of the pelvis, in order that we might give the proper blood flow, or proper flow of blood supply, and through this, and with the condition of the body which is good, as we have given, remove by absorption through the proper channels the conditions and relieve the pains to the head, - not as a special treatment to the head, except just along the cervical on the left side of the body. Keep this up for about six to eight weeks, and we will find we will have a better condition and a balance of force to resist the nervous condition coming to the body, and we will have a proper distribution of all blood and nerve forces in this body here. Do that." (4886-1)

—Radio-Active Device—

As I wrote earlier this device has nothing to do with nuclear energy. It is more like a radio wave device than nuclear fission! The Radio-Active device is mentioned in over 1,000 readings given by Edgar Cayce.

Some people call it the Mind Machine, the BioBattery, the Radial Appliance, the Dry Cell, or the Impedance Device. No batteries and no electrical outlets are involved. To use it, you place it in the sun to "charge" it, Cayce says, then put in a container (pot or bucket), add ice, then add water, wait 15 minutes and attach the connectors to your wrists and ankles in a complex manner which is described in the instruction booklet that comes with it. But all of this information and so much more is on the Edgar Cayce Health Database on EdgarCayce.org.

According to the Cayce readings, the Radio-Active device is not a battery. It works by balancing the body's natural energies, and generates no current itself. Although it was originally called the "Radio-Active" Appliance, it contains no radioactivity. It is constructed of steel, glass, carbon and charcoal in a brass container. It contains no chemicals or toxic materials. It should last for many years, but if you should ever need to dispose of it, no special arrangements are necessary. The appliance seems to work best if used for 4 days in a row, which is one complete cycle. After each period of use, the readings recommend that you take a break from it.

The attachments for the appliance are rotated in a 4-day pattern, one complete cycle. This doesn't require that you use the appliance 4 days in a row but that is a good way to use it.

Edgar Cayce insisted that anything that can be helpful or healing could also be detrimental if misused. Remember that the Radio-Active device merely utilizes the body's own energy – physically, mentally and spiritually. If there is negativity in our hearts and minds, the device will only redistribute the negative effects throughout our bodies. Keep a positive, constructive attitude while using the device. Edgar Cayce frequently recommended that the person using the device be prayerful and meditative during the session. Using positive affirmations is helpful (affirmations are on page 157).

Baar Products sells their version of this device under the name Radiac (pronounced *ray-dee-ack*).

—Violet Ray Device—

The Violet Ray is a high frequency device using a low amperage to produce static electricity. The appliance derives its name from the violet color of the electrical discharge that emanates during use. The device was recommended in over 900 readings for a wide variety of problems requiring a stimulation to the nervous and circulatory systems. It is a Tesla coil named for Nikola Tesla, the electrical engineer, scientist, inventor, and discoverer, who was granted 1,200 patents and is probably best known for his contribution of alternating current. The device consists of a cylindrical base that is held in the hand. A glass vacuum tube in inserted into the end and glows with the violet color. Typically, the violet ray was recommended in conjunction with other therapies such as spinal adjustments. Spinal manipulation was often recommended before beginning the violet ray sessions.

I have used this device on my late wife to help with her healing. Many people put the glass applicator right on the skin before turning the device on and turning it off before removing it from the skin to avoid a static electrical shock (like when you slide your shocking feet on a carpet and then touch a metal door nob - sap, you get a shock. However, in his readings Cayce recommends that you do not contact the skin but run the device above the skin yet not close enough to generate an arcing spark of static electricity, which will give the person a sap!

A pleasant ozone smell and a sizzling noise occur during the use of this device. On the website Cayce.com we have this insight written by healthcare professional Elaine Hruska: "Ozone, a form of oxygen (O3), is produced from the combination of static electricity and the oxygen in the air. Found in the atmosphere in minute quantities, it is the familiar odor detected after a thunderstorm. In some areas it is utilized as an alternative to chlorine in destroying bacteria in the water supply. Cayce in several readings encouraged people to inhale this distinct odor of ozone, stating that it would be beneficial."

You should not have any alcohol in your system during one of these sessions. However, Cayce did recommend ingesting a specific ingredient to enhance the healing.

In several readings he recommended that you ingest a 1/4 teaspoon of animated ash and wait 10 to 15 minutes for the ash to get into the circulatory system, then apply the device. The ash in the circulation will give off oxygen when it comes into region of the body where the violet ray is penetrating, and oxygenation is healthful in improving many conditions. As noted earlier the electrical atmosphere between the skin and the device will generate ions and a very specific scent will fill the air; he wanted the patient to inhale this air for its health benefits.

Much more information and greater detail go to the EdgarCayce.org website (especially the Edgar Cayce Healthcare Database section), Cayce.com, and Baar.com.

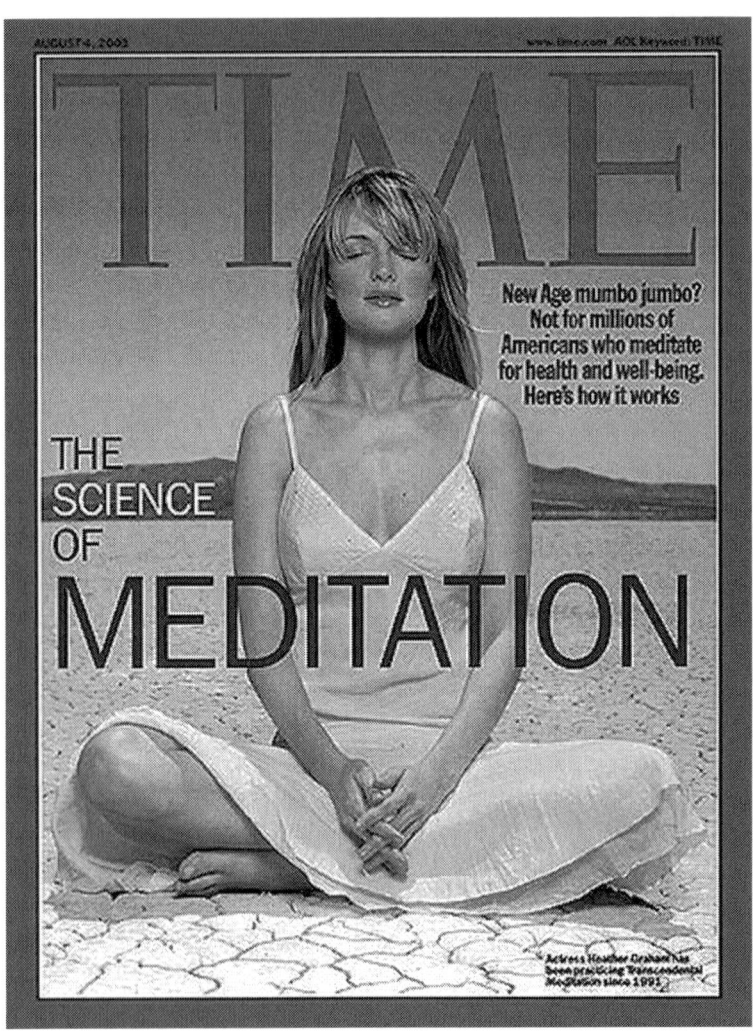

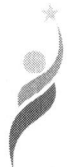

Chapter 9
Metaphysical Concepts and Methods of Healing

—Attunement is Required—

Unique to Cayce's vision is the idea that we seekers of healing and health must attune ourselves to the Divine that is within every cell of our bodies in order to fully realize the perfected condition. It's like a pattern, a code, a vibration of life in its ideal condition. And when we attune to it, we begin to imbue ourselves with this perfected life pattern, this vibration, this state of being.

"It will require that there be such an attitude in mind, in purpose, in hope, and in relationships to others, that each cell of the body may be attuned to the divine within. Each cell must become expectant, that there may be the renewing, the revivifying of the relationships that the soul-entity bears to Creative Forces." (3511-1)

"Thus there may be a revivifying, a resuscitating, a creating of an environment such that the body-mind, with its spiritual concepts and its spiritual understanding, may arouse the whole of the body-forces to their better function-ings." (1620-1)

"For the body mentally, in its spiritual attributes for the physical self, may hold much in this manner – as the applications are made, osteopathically, electrically – not for things to be gotten through with, but SEE, FEEL, KNOW that these are channels and measures through which the divine may operate for effective activity in this body!" (1299-1)

"The addition of energy-building forces has not removed the hurt, the disappointment. For this has attacked the physical body through the sensory and sympathetic nervous system, causing the reaction. Not that there is any mental disturbance, no. It is rather a hurt, an injury, a disappointment such that there can only come the renewing, the revivifying, by putting the whole trust, faith and renewed life in divine hands." (4037-1)

"Being able to raise within the vibrations of individuals to that which is a resuscitating, a revivifying influence and force through the deep meditation (the attunement of self to the higher vibrations in Creative Forces), these are manifested in man through the promises that are coming from Creative Forces or Energy itself!" (993-4)

"Put hope and trust and faith in the divine within – the revivifying, the rejuvenating of that spirit of life and truth within every atom of the body. This will put to flight all of those things that hinder a body from giving expression of the most hopeful, the most beautiful." (572-5)

"There are those forces as may be had from the study, the analyzing of those truths presented in the light of HIS ministry – that One who is the way, the truth and the light. The analyzing of these, and the application of same in the lives of individuals is an individual experience. But the closer, the nearer one applies those tenets, those truths, those principles in one's daily experience, the greater is the ability of the mental and spiritual self to revivify the physical activities of any given body." (2074-1)

"When the Prince of Peace came into the earth for the completing of His OWN development in the earth, HE overcame the flesh AND temptation. So He became the first of those that overcame death in the body, enabling Him to so illuminate, to so revivify that body as to take it up again, even when those fluids of the body had been drained away by the nail holes in His hands and by the spear piercing His side." (1152-1)

—Intuitive Healing & Visualization—

"Intuition – the faculty – is so often misunderstood. Psychic forces and psychic development are so often misunderstood. Psychic should be applied rather to the soul mind or soul body, than merely to (as is the more often deduced) the MENTAL activities...." (255-12)

From Cayce's point of view, a view from the Universal Consciousness, intuition and psychic development are not mental activities. They are soul abilities. In reading 3744-2, Cayce states that psychic activities are the soul's ability to bring these into the physical plane. The outer self has little idea of where these insights or knowings come from, but sees their influence in daily life.

Intuition and psychic knowing do not come from mental activity but from a closer proximity to one's soul forces, soul body. If we seek to grow closer to our soul, we will naturally become more intuitive and psychic.

Ms. 255 asked Cayce specifically for some training. She was not expecting the answer he gave:

"(Q) Suggest how the entity may train self in the present to the study and use of this intuitive sense.

"(A) Train intuition? Then, how would you train electricity – save as to how it may be governed! By keeping in self those thoughts, those activities of the mental mind, those activities of the body that allow spiritual truths to emanate through. Not train, but govern! Govern it by knowing that the mind, that the body, that the influences are such that these are not sidetracked from the ideals and purposes that are set before self. So develop. For God, the Giver of all good and perfect gifts, He who metes to every soul that which is the companionship to its activities in a material life, guards, and guides and keeps those that in sincerity seek to know HIS way, irrespective of the other influences that may be about a body. Hence, in governing, in guarding, in guiding such forces, such powers that arise or manifest or demonstrate through the activities of the body, keep the body, the mind, the soul, in attune with the spheres of celestial forces, rather than of earthly forces." (255-12)

—Tip for Manifesting Desires into Reality—

There has been a lot of talk about the power and importance of visualization in realizing one's desires. But Cayce takes a much different view of this approach.

"(Q): To bring a desired THING or CONDITION into manifestation, is it advisable to visualize it by making a PICTURE or just to hold the idea in prayer and let God produce it in His own way without our making a pattern?

"(A) The pattern is given you in the mount. The MOUNT is within your inner self. To visualize by 'picturizing' is to *bome* [means to celebrate] idol worshipers. Is this pleasing, with your conception of your God that has given, 'Have no other gods before me'? The God in self, the God of the universe, then, meets you in your inner self. Be patient, and leave it with Him. He knows what you have need of before you ask. Visualizing is telling Him how it must look when you have received it. Is that your conception of an All-Wise, All-Merciful Creator? Then, let rather your service ever be, 'Not my will, O God, but Your be done in me, through me.' For all is His. Then, think like it – and, most of all, act like it is." (705-2)

The next question is about healing and keeping healthy the physical by nonphysical means. Cayce's answer seems to indicate that, though this is possible, the physical body ultimately lives in a physical dimension with laws of its own that must be honored.

"(Q) Do you not believe if one can make herself positive to ONLY the GOOD she can overcome all physical ills of the body, without medicine, provided she feeds it right and treats it right?

"(A) What manner of body in a material world can live, survive or remain material without material sustenance? In each sphere of activity there are the attributes. The body-physical may indeed be healed without medicine, but it becomes rather the ethereal than material." (705-2)

Here Cayce is explaining there are physical needs for a physical body, even if she has an ethereal mind she has to attend to the body's physical needs.

—Affirmations—

One of the best practices for manifesting desires is through the use of words and thoughts held in the heart and mind of the one seeking. Cayce called these "affirmations."

"By affirmation, we mean that it should be an AFFIRMATION! Not merely spoken in a singsong manner or said just once. Take at least the time to repeat the affirmation, positively, three to five times that there may be the full, positive response in the mental activities of the body." (271-4)

Of all the wonderful guidance to come through Edgar Cayce's attunement to the Universal Consciousness, using an affirmation to change one's mind, mood, health, perspective, abilities, and reach for new potentials is a unique idea. He gave over a hundred affirmations to people seeking physical, mental, or spiritual help.

From his perspective, an affirmation is an ideal structured in a potently suggestive statement. He instructed us to speak (aloud or silently) the affirmation, being sure to maintain a consciousness of the meaning of the words, and to speak it with a positive, expectant attitude until the whole of our mental being is affected positively by the meaning. He suggested that the affirmation be repeated three to five times, and the goal is to achieve a "full, positive response" from the mental portion of our being.

I have selected three of his affirmations, which are printed at the end of this article. The first one was intended to take hold of desires, needs, and attitudes that we all experience in life and move them to a higher, more universally attuned condition, resulting in greater harmony and happiness in our lives. After shaping this affirmation, Cayce sharply instructed the person to "leave it with Him" rather than to keep wondering and doubting, in anxious waiting for immediate results. He wanted people to feel the power of the affirmation in their mental self and then let it go free. The reason for this, he said, was that the "unseen forces," more powerful than the seen, work in a different way. The unseen forces work best when we have faith in them, a demonstrated faith shown by allowing them to work their magical way through our bodies, minds, hearts, and lives. He said that the spirit of patience, expectancy, and contentment are fertile soil from which the unseen forces can bring forth their miracles.

The second affirmation was designed to help a person find the best ways to be a channel of blessings to others. Cayce explained that the phrase "my going in and my coming out" (taken from Exodus 28:35) is speaking about going in to the Holy Place within us, where God meets with us, and coming out from that Holy Place to interact with others and our outer work. The going in is mostly done during sleep, prayer, meditation, and moments of reflection and stillness.

The third affirmation was designed to connect us with what Cayce called "the Christ Consciousness," a state of mind and perspective that best channels the power of light and love into and through us – an excellent state to be in. If you are not Christian or have had some bad karma with Christianity, in one reading Cayce used the term God-Consciousness as a synonym for Christ-Consciousness. The term Christ is simply the Greek language version of the Hebrew term Messiah. Both literally mean "anointed one." I find it helpful to think of Christ as the personal conscious contact point for each of us within the vast, infinite, impersonal God of the Cosmos. They are one and the same, but the Messiah is that promised direct-connection point that God gave to the prophet Daniel through the archangel Gabriel (the first time the term Messiah appears in the Bible).

In addition to meditation times, affirmations are excellent mantras to use throughout the day, especially when challenges appear or one is feeling down, unhappy, unsure, or stuck. They're also great ways to sing the joys and thanksgivings when life is good!

Let my desire and my needs be in Thy hands, Thou Maker, Creator of the universe and all the forces and powers therein! And may I conform my attitude, my purpose, my desire, to that Thou hast as an activity for me. (Now leave it with Him and go to work!) (462-8)

Lord, here am I! Use Thou me in the ways as Thou knowest best. May my going in and my coming out always be acceptable in Thy sight, my Lord, my Strength, and my Redeemer. (2803-3)

Let that mind be in me that was in Him, who knew that of Himself He could do nothing, yet in the power of the light of the Father of all may we, may I, may all, come to know His love the better. Thy will, O Father, be done in me just now. (436-3)

—Spiritual Healing—

Spiritual healing uses the power of the life forces beyond the physical, material reality to affect a change in the physical body. It uses prayer, meditative attunement to higher forces, to God and the Great Spirit, the Source of all life, and then channels this to the body needing help. It can be done within oneself or through oneself to another. Here are some of Cayce's comments and directives:

"(Q) By what steps are developed the powers of spiritual healing?

"(A) Through spiritual growth. By what powers does a grain of corn maintain its ability to produce corn; that divine gift to the first corn? By not trying to be something other than a grain of corn! Thus may there come an understanding to any soul, to any that will say, 'Use me, O God, as You will.' But not remaining idle! For, as has been given, ACTIVITY IS the key to understanding. For movement is the effect of spirit. Spirit is life. But let the inner self, the divine self, the knowledge of same, be directed only by Him." (705-2)

It sounds so obvious, so simple. When God created us, He/She put His/Her spark of life and health in us. And, as in the grain of corn, we simply have to be the children of God that we are, and life will produce life. Finally, with this concept in our minds and hearts, we must also be up and doing! In actively applying ourselves each day comes the growth of understanding.

We will explore spiritual healing further in the following reading from the Cayce files:

TEXT OF READING 281-24

This psychic reading given by Edgar Cayce at his home on Arctic Crescent, Virginia Beach, Va., this 29th day of June, 1935, in accordance with request made by those present; second reading of the Association Fourth Annual Congress.

PRESENT

Edgar Cayce; Gertrude Cayce, Conductor; Gladys Davis, Steno. Hereward & Marie Sweet Carrington, Gladys & Douglas Johnston, Edith Fox, Josephine L. B. Macsherry, Mae Smith, Edna B. Harrell, Anna E. Hendley, Anne Penn, Florence Edmonds, Esther Wynne, Helen Ellington, Margaret Wilkins, H. E. Poole, Boyd Davis, & others; including L. B. & Hugh Lynn Cayce, Pearl E. Hood, Ethel Libbey and Stella Monsch.

READING

Time of Reading 11:45 to 12:30 A. M.

1. GC: You will have before you the laws of spiritual healing. You will give a discourse at this time on psychic (spiritual) healing, describing just what takes place in the body

and mind of one healed. You will answer the questions that may be presented.

2. : Yes, we have the laws that govern spiritual or psychic healing. Much has been given through these channels from time to time respecting that necessary in the individual experience for healing.

3. As we have indicated, the body-physical is an atomic structure subject to the laws of its environment, its heredity, its SOUL development.

4. The activity of healing, then, is to create or make a balance in the necessary units of the influence or force that is set in motion as the body in the material form, through the motivative force of spiritual activity, sets in motion.

5. It is seen that each atom, each corpuscle, has within same the whole form of the universe - within its OWN structure.

6. As for the PHYSICAL body, this is made up of the elements of the various natures that keep same in its motion necessary for sustaining its equilibrium; as begun from its (the individual body's) first cause.

7. If in the atomic forces there becomes an overbalancing, an injury, a happening, an accident, there are certain atomic forces destroyed or others increased; that to the physical body become either such as to add to or take from the 'elan vitale' that makes for the motivative forces through that particular or individual activity.

8. Then, in meeting these it becomes necessary for the creating of that influence within each individual body to bring a balance necessary for its continued activity about each of the atomic centers its own rotary or creative force, its own elements for the ability of resuscitating, revivifying, such influence or force in the body.

9. How, then, does the activity of ANY influence act upon the individual system for bringing HEALING in the wake or the consciousness, to become conscious of its desire?

10. When a body, separate from that one ill, then, has so attuned or raised its own vibrations sufficiently, it may - by the motion of the spoken word - awaken the activity of the emotions to such an extent as to revivify, resuscitate or to change the rotary force or influence or the atomic forces in the activity of the structural portion, or the *vitale* forces of a body, in such a way and manner as to set it again in motion.

11. Thus does spiritual or psychic influence of body upon body bring healing to ANY individual; where another body may raise that necessary influence in the hormone of the circulatory forces as to take from that within itself to revivify or resuscitate diseased, disordered or distressed conditions within a body.

12. For, as has been said oft, any manner in which healing comes - whether by the laying on of hands, prayer, by a look, by the application of any mechanical influence or any of those forces in *materia medica* - must be of such a nature as to produce that necessary within those forces about the atomic centers of a given body for it to bring resuscitating or healing.

13. The law, then, is compliance with the universal spiritual influence that awakens any atomic center to the necessity of its concurrent activity in relationships to other pathological forces or influences within a given body. Whether this is by spiritual forces, by any of the mechanical forces, it is of necessity one and the same. Many are the divisions or characters of those ills that befall or become a portion of each individual body. Some are set in motion so that certain portions of the glandular system or of the organs of the body perform more than their share. Hence some are thin, some are fat, some are tall, some are short.

14. What said He? Can anyone by taking thought make one hair white or black, or add one cubit to his stature? WHO giveth healing, then?

15. It is in any manner the result only of compliance to the First Cause, and the activity of same within the individual's RELATIVE relation to its own evolution.

16. Ready for questions.

17. (Q) Is group action more effective than individual, and if so why? (A) "Where two or three are gathered in my name, I am in the midst of them." These words were spoken by Life, Light, Immortality, and are based on a law. For, in union is strength. Why?

Because as there is oneness of purpose, oneness of desire, it becomes motivative within the active forces or influences of a body. The multiplicity of ideas may make confusion, but added cords of strength in one become of the nature as to increase the ABILITY and influence in every expression of such a law.

18. (Q) In any form of psychic healing, is an etheric intermediary employed? (A) Possible; but the etheric body of the individual seeking or finding expression must be in accord with that which draws upon such an influence.

19. (Q) In certain types of insanity, is there an etheric body involved? If so, how? (A) Possession.

Let's for a moment use examples that may show what has oft been expressed from here:

There is the physical body, there is the mental body, there is the soul body. They are One, as the Trinity; yet these may find a manner of expression that is individual unto themselves. The body itself finds its own level in its OWN development. The mind, through anger, may make the body do that which is contrary to the better influences of same; it may make for a change in its environ, its surrounding, contrary to the laws of environment or hereditary forces that are a portion of the 'elan vitale' of each manifested body, with the spirit or the soul of the individual.

Then, through pressure upon some portion of the anatomical structure that would make for the disengaging of the natural flow of the mental body through the physical in its relationships to the soul influence, one may be dispossessed of the mind; thus ye say rightly he is "out of his mind."

Or, where there are certain types or characters of disease found in various portions of the body, there is the lack of the necessary 'vitale' for the resuscitating of the energies that carry on through brain structural forces of a given body. Thus disintegration is produced, and ye call it dementia praecox - by the very smoothing of the indentations necessary for the rotary influence or vital force of the spirit within same to find expression. Thus derangements come.

Such, then, become possessed as of hearing voices, because of their closeness to the Borderland. Many of these are termed deranged when they may have more of a closeness to the universal than one who may be standing nearby and commenting; yet they are awry when it comes to being normally balanced or healthy for their activity in a material world.

"(Q) Is it possible to give any advice as to how an individual may raise his own vibrations, or whatever may be necessary, to effect a self-cure?

"(A) By raising that attunement of self to the spirit within, that is of the soul - body - about which we have been speaking.

"Oft in those conditions where necessary ye have seen produced within a body unusual or abnormal strength, either for physical or mental activity. From whence arose such? WHO hath given you power? Within what live ye? WHAT is Life? Is it the ATTUNING of self, then, to same. HOW?

"As the body-physical is purified, as the mental body is made wholly at-one with purification or purity, with the life and light within itself, healing comes, strength comes, power comes.

"So may an individual effect a healing, through meditation, through attuning not just a side of the mind nor a portion of the body but the whole, to that at-oneness with the spiritual forces within, the gift of the life-force within each body.

"For (aside, please), when matter comes into being, what has taken place? The Spirit ye worship as God has MOVED in space and in time to make for that which gives its expression; perhaps as wheat, as corn, as flesh, as whatever may be the movement in that ye call time and space.

"Then MAKING self in an at-onement with that Creative Force brings what? That necessary for the activity which has been set in motion and has become manifested to be in accord WITH that First Cause.

"Hence do we find it becomes necessary that ye speak, ye act, that way. For whosoever cometh to offer to self, or to make an offering to the throne of mercy or grace, and speaks unkind of his brother, is only partially awake or aware.

"For that which has brought distraughtness, distress, disease in the earth, or in manifestation, is transgression of the law.

"We are through for the present."??

—Aspects of Our Being
And How to Know Them—

In the Edgar Cayce vision we are more than physical beings with material bodies, and learning more about our whole makeup is helpful to health and healing.

Here is a Cayce discourse on that will add to our understanding. It begins with the suggest and then Cayce responds:

"You will have before you the body and enquiring mind of [2475], ..., Penna., in special reference to the Yoga exercises with which he has been experimenting, in breathing. You will indicate just what has taken place in the body and what should be done from this point, considering the best physical, mental and spiritual development of the entity. You will answer the questions, as I ask them:

"Yes, we have the body, the enquiring mind, [2475]; and those conditions, those experiences of the body in the use of Yoga exercise in breathing.

To give that as would be helpful to the body at this time, there might be indicated for the body something of that which takes place when such exercises are used - and the experiences had by one so doing.

"These exercises are excellent, yet it is necessary that special preparation be made - or that a perfect understanding be had by the body as to what takes place when such exercises are used.

"For, BREATH is the basis of the living organism's activity. Thus, such exercises may be beneficial or detrimental in their effect upon a body.

"Hence it is necessary that an understanding be had as to how, as to when, or in what manner such may be used.

"It would be very well for the body to study very carefully the information which we have given through these sources as respecting Meditation. Then this information as may be given here may prove of beneficial effect in the experience of the body.

"Each soul, individual or entity, finds these facts existent:

"There is the body-physical - with all its attributes for the functioning of the body in a three-dimensional or a manifested earth plane.

"Also there is the body-mental - which is that directing influence of the physical, the mental and the spiritual emotions and manifestations of the body; or the way, the manner in which conduct is related to self, to individuals, as well as to things, conditions and circumstances. While the mind may not be seen by the physical senses, it can be sensed by others; that is, others may sense the conclusions that have been drawn by the body-mind of an individual, by the manner in which such an individual conducts himself in relationship to things, conditions or people.

"Then there is the body-spiritual, or soul-body - that eternal something that is invisible. It is only visible to that consciousness in which the individual entity in patience becomes aware of its relationship to the mental and the physical being.

"All of these then are one - in an entity; just as it is considered, realized or acknowledged that the body, mind and soul are one, - that God, the Son and the Holy Spirit are one.

"Then in the physical body there ARE those influences, then, through which each of these phases of an entity may or does become an active influence.

"There may be brought about an awareness of this by the exercising of the mind, through the manner of directing the breathing.

"For, in the body there is that center in which the soul is expressive, creative in its nature, - the Leydig center.

"By this breathing, this may be made to expand - as it moves along the path that is taken in its first inception, at conception, and opens the seven centers of the body that radiate or are active upon the organisms of the body.

"This in its direction may be held or made to be a helpful influence for specific conditions, at times - by those who have taught, or who through experience have found as it were the key, or that which one may do and yet must not do; owing to whatever preparation has been made or may be made by the body for the use of this ability, this expression through the body-forces.

"As this life-force is expanded, it moves first from the Leydig center through the adrenals, in what may be termed an upward trend, to the pineal and to the centers in control of the emotions - or reflexes through the nerve forces of the body.

"Thus an entity puts itself, through such an activity, into association or in conjunction with all it has EVER been or may be. For, it loosens the physical consciousness to the universal consciousness.

167

"To allow self in a universal state to be controlled, or to be dominated, may become harmful.

"But to know, to feel, to comprehend as to WHO or as to WHAT is the directing influence when the self-consciousness has been released and the real ego allowed to rise to expression, is to be in that state of the universal consciousness, - which is indicated in this body here, Edgar Cayce, through which there is given this interpretation for [2475's name was here].

"So, in analyzing all this, - first study the variations of what has been the body-temperament, in thought, in food. For, the body-physical becomes that which it assimilates from material nature. The body-mental becomes that it assimilates from both the physical-mental and the spiritual-mental. The soul is ALL of that the entity is, has been or may be.

"Then, WHO and WHAT would the entity have to direct self in such experiences?

"To be loosed without a governor, or a director, may easily become harmful.

"But as we would give, from here, let not such a director be that of an entity. Rather so surround self with the universal consciousness of the CHRIST, as to be directed by that influence as may be committed to you.

"Thus the entity may use constructively that which has been attained.

"But to prevent physical harm, mental harm, - attune self in body and in mind with that influence by which the entity seeks to be directed; not haphazardly, not by chance, but - as of old - choose you this day WHOM ye will serve: the living God within you, by you, through you? or those influences of knowledge without wisdom, that would enslave or empower you with the material things which only gratify for the moment?

"Rather choose you as he of old, - let others do as they may, but as for you, serve you the living God.

Thus ye may constructively use that ability of spiritual attunement, which is the birthright of each soul; ye may use it as a helpful influence in your experiences in the earth.

"But make haste SLOWLY! Prepare the body. Prepare the mind, before ye attempt to loosen it in such measures or manners that it may be taken hold upon by those influences which constantly seek expressions of self rather than of a living, constructive influence of a CRUCIFIED Savior.

"Then, crucify desire in self; that ye may be awakened to the real abilities of helpfulness that lie within your grasp.

"Ready for questions.

"(Q) Is there at present any danger to any particular body function, such as sex; or to general health?

"(A) As we have indicated, without preparation, desires of EVERY nature may become so accentuated as to destroy - or to overexercise as to bring detrimental forces; unless the desire and purpose is acknowledged and set IN the influence of self as to its direction - when loosened by the kundaline activities through the body.

"(Q) Just what preparation would you advise for the body, now?

"(A) This should be rather the choice of the body from its OWN development, than from what ANY other individual entity or source might give.

"Purify the body, purify the mind; that the principle, the choice of ideals as made by the entity may be made manifest.

"Do whatever is required for this, - whether the washing of the body, the surrounding with this or that influence, or that of whatever nature.

"As has been experienced, this opening of the centers or the characters of breathing, - for, as indicated, the breath is power in itself; and this power may be directed to certain portions of the body. But for what purpose? As yet it has been only to see what will happen! Remember what curiosity did to the cat! Remember what curiosity did to Galileo, and what it did to Watt - but they used it in quite different directions in each case!

"(Q) Considering the development of the entity, is further practice of the Yoga exercises of breathing and meditation recommended?

"(A) By all means! if and when, and ONLY when, preparation has been made; and when there is the knowledge, the understanding and the wisdom as to what to do WITH that gained! Without such, do not undertake same!

"We are through for the present." (2475-1)

—Dreams and Meditation—

Two practices consistently recommended by Cayce to develop and include in our lives were the benefits of a dream life and meditation practice. And he considered these to also of much help in healing, health, and rejuvenation.

—Dreams—

Sleep research centers have proven that everyone dreams, every night! The sleep state called REM (for Rapid Eye Movement) is a necessary phase of a night's sleep, and it is during this stage that the researchers wake people and find that all of them are dreaming. The challenge is to bring the memory of that dream into the outer, daily consciousness.

Edgar Cayce considered the activity of the mind during dreams and visions to be important to developing one's whole development. Here's one of his comments:

"The dreams, as we see, come to the entity through those channels as have been outlined for the entity, and are for the entity's edification, will they (the dreams) be but applied in the physical or material life, for the dreams and visions are as experiences to the mental forces, and the mental or mind is the Builder." (137-92)

It is important to record our dreams and interpret them, comprehend them, or at least get the gist of them. Such understanding would bring a bigger vision of life to the outer person than could be gained with only outer study and application. Dreams, he said, can bring warnings and opportunities that would otherwise be lost. In fact, he said that nothing occurs in our life that is not first foreshadowed in our dreams! A journal beside the bed is his recommendation, though some of us have successfully used tape recorders (not a good idea if you sleep with someone—too noisy).

What are dreams? Cayce answers: "Dreams are of different natures, and have their inception from influences either in the body, in the mind, or from the realm of the soul and spirit."

Here's another of his comments: "Dreams are of many natures. Dreams, as we have given, are either from the material activity of individual influences attempting to be assimilated, or warring with those influences within the body, and bring visions or experiences that are at times called nightmares, night horses or the like. Those are experiences also through which the subconscious forces are constantly aware of what has been the experience, and it comes as an influence for foreseeing or for premonition or experiences. And necessarily unless they are impressed more than once become rather as dreams. Then there are experiences of the soul that has been awakened to the knowledge which has been or may be written upon same, the experiences of the entity as an entity through its sojourns - and these are given then in emblems or in visions that are to be and are a part of the individual entity. Such became the case here. In the meeting of same, trust in Him who IS the power, who IS the strength, and abide by His judgments - not yours." (281-27)

One of the first steps toward interpretation of a dream is to identify what is the influence behind the dream: Is it the body, the mind, or the soul?

Cayce says that the most common influence impelling dreams is "mental development." Our subconscious (mind of our soul) and our superconscious (mind of our godly self) are attempting to correlate life events and decisions with eternal, spiritual ideals and purposes. On one occasion Cayce modified the word correlation to "co-relation of subconscious and superconscious forces manifesting through the developing mind of the entity." Generally, the feeling or mood that accompanies the dream reveals how our deeper soul-life feels about the outer-life events, decisions, and conditions.

Beyond the common correlating process, some dreams are about conditions in the body that need to be cared for; some deal with opportunities that need to be seized or situations that need to be avoided; others are non-physical experiences in other dimensions of life that help us expand our consciousness. In some dreams we break the time barrier and see far into the past or into the future. The subconscious mind is like a bird high above the road we are traveling; it can see around the next bend on our path and review the distant roads we've traveled and forgotten.

Dreams are multidimensional. It is this very quality that makes them so difficult to understand. They have a language all their own; a language of imagery, symbolism, and sometimes bizarre activity. As all who have studied their dreams can attest, dreams are often difficult to interpret and understand. And yet, many humans have received life-changing insight and guidance through dreams, even major inventions have been as a result of dream. From biblical journeys with God to modern scientific breakthroughs, dreams have played a major role in the human experience.

—How to Remember Dreams—

Before we get into the nature of dreams, let's review some good tips for *remembering* them. It is often difficult for us to keep from jumping out of sleep into our outer, earthly minds and its business, but getting the dream from the deeper is the first step in adding dream value to our lives.

Edgar Cayce recommends three simple things:

1. Give yourself a pre-sleep suggestion;
2. Don't move the body upon waking;

3. Record the content or impressions right away.

When we are "falling asleep," as we like to call it, we are actually moving from our outer conscious mind to our inner subconscious. The subconscious is always amenable to suggestion (one of the keys to hypnosis). If, as we are entering the subconscious, we are repeating a suggestion to remember our dreams, the subconscious takes that suggestion to heart. However, the body is mostly physical and if we move it too quickly upon waking, we will jump straight out of our subconscious into our outer daily consciousness and lose the dream. Therefore, we must resist moving the body upon waking. Linger in the twilight, between the outer mind and the inner—or, as the Egyptians described it: between the land of the living and the land of the dead (sleep is the shadow of death). Here we will find our dream content and imagery.

—How to Interpret Dreams—

When it comes to interpretation, Cayce always said that the best interpreter of the dream is the dreamer: "You interpret dreams in yourself. Not by a dream book, not by what others say, but dreams are presented in symbols, in signs." It is important to recognize that the dreamer is our inner self. Therefore, the best interpreter is our inner self, so we should obtain the interpretation while still in or near the dreaming self. Trying to translate a dream later with only our outer, three-dimensional self is very difficult. It did not dream the dream. We will do much better if we keep the body and outer self still as we awaken, and get the dream and its meaning from the inner self.

Here are some quick steps toward better interpretation:

1. Watch your mood upon waking. This will give you the best sense of whether the inner self is happy or unhappy about conditions.

2. Get the gist of the dream first, details second. Jesus once observed that we tend to strain for gnats while we are swallowing camels. (Matthew 23:24) The big picture, the

173

overriding *theme*, is much more important for us to grasp than the details.

3. Understand that the subconscious may use exaggeration to get our attention. It's like the joke of how to get your mule to do something: first, you hit him as hard as you can to get his attention. In a similar manner the subconscious gets our attention: exaggerated activities and shocking imagery will do more to get our attention than sweetly whispered instructions. Therefore, don't let the dramatic exaggerations overwhelm you or cause fear. In fact, the bizarre image or activity is likely the key to interpreting the entire dream.

4. Dreams are usually symbolic. They speak in imagery that represents more than literal appearance. Like good parables or novelettes, they tell a story that has a deeper meaning than the details. Often they use figures of speech. For example, if I told you that I really put my foot in my mouth while talking with someone yesterday, you would know that I did not literally put my foot in my mouth. Dreams speak in the same manner and are best interpreted as you would figures of speech.

5. Finally, nothing will help us get better dream guidance than using dream content in our lives. Create an action plan for each dream. Ask yourself, How can I use this dream in my life today? Even if you are not really sure of the dream's meaning, attempt to use some portion of it. In this way your inner self will be stimulated to bring more insight and guidance through the dream channel, and it will become clearer and more relevant.

Budget time for dream recall and interpretation, because dreams guide us to the shores of paradise. Sleep is a shadow of death and the life beyond this world. To live in dreamy sleep is to know the heavens beyond this world.

—**Edgar Cayce State of Consciousness**—

Let's consider Cayce's state of mind during his psychic condition. Here are some details coming from his readings about him giving these strange discourses.

"Yes, we have that work as manifests itself through the body Edgar Cayce, and the enquiring minds of those present in this room. Ready for questions.

"(Q) What caused the extraordinary physical reaction with Edgar Cayce at the close of the reading [254-67] this morning, at the beginning of the suggestion?

"(A) As was seen, through the seeking of irrelevant questions there was antagonism manifested. This made for a contraction of those channels through which the activity of the psychic forces operates in the material body; as we have outlined, along the pineal, the lyden [cells of Leydig] and the [spinal] cord—or silver cord. The natural reactions are for sudden contraction when changing suddenly from the mental-spiritual to material.

"For, as evidenced by that which has been given, there is the touching—with the mental beings of those present in the room or at such manifestations—of the most delicate mechanism that may be well imagined.

"As has been crudely given, a hen may lay an egg but the shell once cracked or broken CANNOT be made to produce that it contains.

"When the thought, the activity that is being made manifest, is broken, that which is creative or constructive— once touched by thought or suggestion—is hindered, wavered, as to that it may bring to a manifested form.

"Hence the experiences that are sometimes held, or that may be held, by those that may witness or experience the transmission of that which is received or gained through this particular channel, may—by the mere disturbing of the body that rests above the natural body by other than the elements that have not taken bodily form—break the associations, the connections, with that source from which the records are being taken.

"In considering such information, much—and much more—might be given, or sought, as to how far-reaching in space (time) is the information or the effects or benefits from such reaching, in its range or scope of activity.

"As has been demonstrated by the parallel drawn respecting how the channel or medium operates in the relationships to the manners of transmission of a sense-consciousness, as through the radio, this depends only upon the manner of the transformer or the attunement and that which may interfere that is of the characterized element which indicates the channel of transmission through which the reception may come.

"This, in the physical sense, has been covered. Many phases of those conditions that influence same, that surround the body, have been touched upon. These might be expanded; though, digest—my brethren—that ye have in hand.

"(Q) What is the significance of the experience had during reading [373-2] Wednesday afternoon, July 12th, in which Edgar Cayce saw himself traveling through water in a bubble and arriving at the place where he always gets the information —the old man with the books?

"(A) To bring from one realm to another those experiences through which an entity, a soul, may pass in obtaining those reflections that are necessary for transmission of the information sought, it becomes necessary (for the understanding of those in that realm seeking) to have that which is to the mental being put in the language of that being, as near as it is possible to do justice to the subject.

"In this particular instance, then, to reach that record suggested by the suggestion itself—as of coming into existence across waters, the very thought of those present that it becomes necessary that that which is to receive or transmit the information must seek (as indicated by the manner in which periods, ages, dates, years, days are turned back, in arriving at the experience of the entity in a changed environ); meant that, the psychic influences in their activity with or through the physical forces of the body, must in some manner pass through the necessary elements for arriving at or reaching the beginning or that point. With the amount of water that is more often thought than of ether, what more befitting than that in the bubble the seeking forces should guide themselves!

"Then, so becomes much that arrives in the material plane; in the form of pictures or expressions, that there may be the conveying to the mind of the seeker something in his own type of experience, as to how the transmission of the activity takes place. Of what forces? The psychic or soul forces, that are akin to what? The Creative Forces, or that called God.

"So, the body in a symbolized form as the bubble arrives at a place in which there is kept the records of all; as signified in speaking of the Book of Life, or to indicate or symbolize that each entity, each soul in its growth, may find its way back to the Creative Influences that are promised in and through Him that gives—and is—Life; and finds this as a separate, a definite, an integral part of the very soul.

"Hence symbolized as being in books; and the man the keeper, as the keeper of the records. Much in the manner as would be said the lord of the storm, of the sea, of the lightning, of the light, of the day, of love, of hope, of faith, of charity, of long-suffering, of brotherly love, of kindness, of meekness, of humbleness, of self.

"So, in the materializations for the concept of those that seek to know, to be enlightened: To the world, long has there been sought that as in books. To many the question naturally arises, then: Are there literally books? To a mind that thinks books, literally BOOKS! As it would be for the mind that in its passage from the material plane into rest would require Elysian fields with birds, with flowers; it must find the materialized form of that portion of the Maker in that realm wherein that entity, that soul, would enjoy such in THAT sphere of activity. As houses built in wood. Wood, in its essence, as given, is what? Books, in their essence, are what? What is the more real, the book with its printed pages, its gilt edges, or the essence of that told of in the book? Which is the more real, the love manifested in the Son, the Savior, for His brethren, or the essence of love that may be seen even in the vilest of passion? They are one. But that they bring into being in a materialized form is what elements of the one source have been combined to produce a materialization. Beautiful, isn't it?

"How far, then, is ungodliness from godliness? Just under, that's all!

"Seek then, ye, in understanding as to where, why, from what source, there may be gained the experiences of an entity, a soul, through its journeys in this the odic sphere, or through that known as this solar system. Each portion of that one whole, in that we call life, as it uses the attributes of the physical forces of a created form manifested in a material world, makes a record; as truly as is seen in the cylinder of the plate of the phonograph, or as is given to the radio transmitter upon the ethers of a material world. Going out where? Only those become conscious of same that have attuned themselves to that which is in accord, or seeking to know—then—His will; for each soul, every soul, should seek to attune its mind, its soul—yea, its body-vibrations—to that He, the Son of man, the Mother-God in Jesus the Christ, lived in the earth. Tune into that light, and it becomes BEAUTIFUL; in that you think, that you are, that you live!

"Then KNOW, by doing, by being, even as He, that "My Spirit bears witness with thy spirit" that ye are indeed, in truth, the sons [and daughters] of a living God who day by day utters speech, night unto night shows knowledge.

"The line has gone out into that we call space, and how have you looked as to where that line would fall? One with

Him, to be guided by Him, or to the aggrandizing of those petty jealousies, those petty hatreds that arise from slights, from slurs in your daily life. What! Will ye allow self to separate self, the real self, from the living Christ? HE calls ever, "If ye love me, keep my commandments." What are His commandments? "Love one another." Do good, speak gently, even to those that you in your darkness of heart feel would do you an injustice.

"With this line, as one sees the manifestations of the acts of man in the earth, man claiming God as the father, the Christ as the elder brother, the patriarchs as teachers and directors, and yet find fault with someone that is less gifted with the Light of His love. Suppose, for the moment, that God looked on your own heart as you have often looked on your brother's life? OBLIVION, incomparable to the mind even of man—even as space or time. THINK—THINK—on these things!

"(Q) Please explain the experience he had Tuesday night, August 29th, while giving Norfolk Group #2 reading [397-1] regarding the marvelous light; tones of individuals merging with the whole, ending with baby at mother's breast.

"(A) As may be easily surmised, as may be known by all who would think well on that which has been given, as to how God in His mercy, in His glory, makes Himself known to His creatures in the earth!

"Think not that the snail or the dragonfly, as he crawls from his slime, does not glorify his Maker. And as he mounts on his wings of gossamer, he fills that place for which he has been—in his realm of activity—designated; in his field, his manner of showing forth his love as manifested from the Creator in the materialized world.

"Man alone, of all His kingdom, abuses the gifts that have been made his through the love that the Father would show, in that he (man) might be a companion, one with Him; not the whole, yet equal to the whole, able in that realm to

179

magnify, glorify, even as the dragon fly, that love the Father bestowed upon His sons.

"Then, when there are those periods when body and mind of a group are in accord, seeking that light, it may be shown unto them that they the more may magnify, glorify, that manifestation of the Father-Son love into the earth.

"Occasionally, as there comes—with the visions of those that enter in—that which has been promised, that they in their activity may be enjoined as one to another in bringing to the earth a manifested glory of those that have gathered, do gather, about the Throne; hence, as He is light, all light, so did the light of the seekers make the way that there might be shown that His promises are sure, that there may come that life in a manifested form that would begin again those of face to face may they speak with the Father and with the Son. [See 3976-15 indicating John the beloved had been Jacob.]

"As is exemplified in the breast, that marked as that that should be the one to nourish a life that would bring into that materialized form, if there will remain those associations, those connections that have been given may make the attunement of a manifestation of a portion of life in a material plane.

"Blessed, then, are they that make their wills one in accord with Him, as they seek to know, "Lord, what would you have me do!" Not Lord, may I do this or that! Show forth, ye all, the Lord's death—DEATH—till He come again, in the lightening of the way for those that seek, those that seek to know His way.

"Even as the child, the breast, meant a growth; so feed ye 'my lambs' [John 21:15-17], that they grow in the nurture, the admonition of THE Lord, the Christ Child.

"(Q) Please explain the experience the next morning, Aug. 30th, while giving [257] business reading [257-119], in which he was going through—and surrounded by—blackness?

"(A) A razor is a wonderful instrument for shaving beards. It will trim pencils, but not many beards after—if used very long.

"A pearl is an adornment, a thing of beauty, created through the irritation of that which manifests itself in a lowly way to those that consider themselves of high estate; but by the very act of irritation to its own vibration is the higher vibration created, or brings about the pearl of great price. Yet it does not look well in the sow's ear.

"In the use then to which, through which, the soul of the body would pass to seek that as may be sought by the varied creations of man's activity in a material life, to what depths must such a soul oft descend to bring back that that may even lend an air of help to a hungry soul?

"Through such irritation, though, oft does the soul grow, even as the pearl. So long as that manifested, then, by the life in a manifested form, keeps pure, little harm may come. But once lost can never be regained; even as that given into the heart of every mother to carry to her chosen one the bloom of life itself—only once!

"So, in the understanding of that as happens when through the shadows or the slime, through the darkness or through the grime, may the soul seek to bring to light that which will ease the burden of a hungry soul, it finds its hardships—yes, here and there; yet may he lead that soul to the heavenly stair! [4/16/34 See 257-130, Par. R1, R5 for similar dreams by EC & [257].]

"(Q) [Submitted by Rev. Thos. D. Wesley Presbyterian minister]: What, where or how is the direct and immediate point of contact between the Personal God and the soul, of which contact the soul is conscious and certain?

"(A) As the sons and daughters of God are personal, are individual, with their many attributes that are characteristics, personalities or individualities, so (as this then is a shadow from that from which it sprang, its Maker) must the Maker be individual, with its attributes and its personalities. And yet fill all of life as becomes manifested in the spiritual realm, the realm of the soul or the temporal house, the abode of the soul for a day.

"As the soul seeks, then, for that which is the sustenance of the body—as what the food is to a developing, a growing body, so are the words of truth (which are life, which are love, which are God) sought that make for growth, even as the digesting of the material things in a body make for a growth. This growth may not be felt in the consciousness of materialization. It is experienced by the consciousness of the soul, by which it enables the soul to use the attributes of the soul's food, even as the growth of the body makes for the use of the muscular forces or attributes of the physical body.

"Where is the contact?

"As ye seek Him, so does like beget like. For, ye are co-laborers with Him, if ye have put on the whole of His love in your own life.

"Feed, then, upon the fruits of the spirit. Love, hope, joy, mercy, long-suffering, brotherly love, and the contact, the growth, will be seen; and within the consciousness of the soul will the awareness come of the personality of the God in thee!

"We are through for the present." (254-68)

—Watch Cayce Interpret Dreams—

The following are dreams by various individuals that were brought to Edgar Cayce and that contain insights into the mind and thoughts. These dreams were interpreted through Cayce's readings while he was in a meditative trance. Watching him interpret dreams is quite helpful in developing our skills with dream interpretation.

"(Q) Monday, November 2, 1925, at home. [Dream:] I was in discussion with [137]. I remember only a portion of this. Recall and interpret and explain to me so that my mind may grasp the significance and I may better understand the lesson intended. That I recall is as follows: Talking to [137], I said:

'Now, [137], you see, death is not the grave as many people think—It is another phenomenized form of life.'

"(A) In this, we find the subconscious forces giving to the conscious mind, in this *emblematical conversation*, those experiences in which the conscious mind may gain the lessons pertaining to the psychology of mental forces, see? The portions as we see given and brought to the consciousness of the entity then, being the crux of that thought as was seen in conversation. This as the conversation, as we gain here: The discussion regarding that seen by the life in an individual and the taking of same by any sudden action, see? and the discussion went into the particular conditions regarding individuals' lives that were taken in heat of passion, or in war, and as the mental developed in discussion, we find the entity sees then in same something of that suggestion as was placed by one, Ballentine (?), in the discussion of life after death. And the entity then sees, through the subconscious forces, that death is as but the beginning of another form of phenomenized [sic] force in the earth's plane, and may not be understood by the third dimension mind from third dimension analysis, but must be seen from that fourth-dimension force as may be experienced by an entity gaining the access to same, by development in the physical plane through the mental processes of an entity. The mind is being correlated with subconscious and spiritual forces that magnify same to the conscious force of an entity in such a manner as said entity gains the insight and concept of such phenomenized conditions, see?

"We see in the physical world the condition in every form of life. As is taken here: We find in a grain of corn or wheat that germ that, set in motion through its natural process with Mother Earth and the elements about same, brings forth corn AFTER ITS KIND, see? the kind and the germ being of a spiritual nature, the husk or corn, and the nature or physical condition, being physical forces, see? Then, as the corn dies, the process is as the growth is seen in that as expressed to the entity, and the entity expressing same, see—that death, as commonly viewed, is not that of the passing away, or becoming a non-entity, but the phenomenized condition in a physical world that may be understood with such an illustration, viewed from the fourth-dimension viewpoint or standpoint, see?" (136-18)

In the following dream-interpretation reading, it helps to recall that all names were replaced with numbers to maintain privacy, and to know that 106 is the mother of two sons, 900 and 137. Her brother, the uncle to her two sons is 91. "GC" is Gertrude Cayce, Edgar's wife, acting as the conductor of the reading session.

"GC: You will have before you the body and the enquiring mind of [106] of New Jersey, and the dream the body had on the morning of June 22, 1925, while asleep in her home. You will give the full interpretation and lesson that is to be gained from this, and you will then answer the questions regarding same as I ask them of you. The dream was: I saw my son, [900], standing by a fire escape window, and he called me over, and as I approached, I saw the fire escape. [900] said to me, 'Ma, I have something to tell you.' 'Is it bad news?' I asked anxiously. 'My uncle is very sick,' [900] answered. 'You mean [91],' I asked eagerly. Then I awakened."

"EC: Yes, we have the enquiring mind and the dream as had by [106], early morning, June 22, 1925.

"As to the interpretation and lessons to be gained from and through this, again we have that projection of the subconscious forces as are manifested through the study and impressions through suggestions carried to same from conscious thought, manifested in the subconscious when the conscious is subjugated, as at this time, and again we find these being capable of being brought to the consciousness. For they have each their meaning and are the projections as were seen in others that have come to the consciousness of this entity.

"In the approach of the body, [900], to the body, [106], we find that union in thought as is brought from the conscious to the subconscious. And as to the escape, this manifesting then the manner in which certain conditions, as are shown, may be overcome. The approach we find being the oneness of thought and intent and purport, that must be in each for the better conduct, element of assistance that may be reached through either.

"With the vision as is told through the body, we see that approach of those surroundings that come close to the mental forces of the body, yet may be reached only through the mental forces in such conditions through that study, through that mind, through that understanding as is reached through that of [900].

"Then, the lesson that one is to gain, this entity, is that through this study there may come the escape from many physical conditions that would mar or cause physical distress to any that surround the mental forces (in physical, see?) of this body.

"Well, then, that much of this be understood, that the greater assistance may be accorded to others through the study and propagation of such phenomena becoming manifest in the mental forces of the body, through the thought as reached by suggestion to the conscious, and this reaching the subconscious in the subjugation of consciousness.

"This, then, gives that the body, the uncle of [900], is ill— ill unto that wherein it might be hard for the escape from the vicissitudes that might be brought through such illness. Yet help, assistance, might be reached through the efforts of that one approaching and giving the information necessary for the knowledge of same to reach the consciousness of this body [106].

"Then, as to how to use same, let those regular channels, as have been begun, be opened for the help that may be given. Well that the body be there in person, see?

"(Q) Well that [106] should be with the brother?

"(A) Very shortly, yes.

"(Q) Does this mean [91] is seriously sick?

"(A) Seriously sick. Not showing as yet, however, in that condition that may come—later, see?

"(Q) What should be done? What can [106] and her son [900] do?

"(A) Offer assistance.

"(Q) Why was the message conveyed to her through her son, [900]?

"(A) For through such channels has the interest of such phenomena become manifested to the body. And only through that approach may same become that manifestation in the manner as would be fully acceptable to the understanding of the mind, [106].

"(Q) Did [900]'s vision of his grandmother in anguish, had quite sometime ago, have anything in relation to this dream of [106]?

"(A) Each and every condition as was given in that has its relation one with the other. The same as we have the projection of conditions in the mental forces of [137] in regard to same condition. For this becomes a projection to the mind of [137]. This became a projection to the spiritual forces as manifest in the superconscious forces to the mind of [900] through other channels. One was direct. One was indirect. Through the manifestations, through the subconscious forces, there was the projecting to the superconscious. The other was the superconscious projection to the subconscious forces in [900] as given.

"(Q) [106]'s other son, [137], saw in psychic condition this sickness of his uncle. [900] saw his grandmother in anguish.

[106] had the above dream. Explain this phenomena in the light of [900]'s understanding of the spiritual forces.

"(A) This has just been given in how the projection of each comes, or is presented to reach the consciousness of each individual. As in this: In that of [137] we find the laying aside of the consciousness, the subconscious projection into that of the superconscious forces, again through suggestion, as is reached or as is wafted by the allowing of the self to become submerged to these conditions. This projection we find bringing then to the consciousness a condition that is to exist, as judged from physical forces. Then a future.

"In that we find in [900], the projection from the superconscious forces in that of the anguish as seen in the grandmother, from the superconscious to the subconscious, and brought to consciousness in the mind of [900].

"In that of the mother, [106], we find the projection through the consciousness to the subconscious and reaching to the consciousness from subconscious projection as an existent condition, each entering then all three phases of the manifestation of a spiritual law, as is seen in the material world and understood from each and by each, according to their understanding and application, or ability of application of this law in the material force or world.

"(Q) What part has the entity, Pauline [...], played in this, in relation to manifestation of [137], of vision of [900], or dream of [106]?

"(A) Only that of the intense desire for help through each source, and the source or force in thought making in a physical, or seeking a physical action, finds its answer in each, through the channels as given. Truly then do thoughts become the deeds, and find, as in this, the manifestation in the different manners in the life of each. As in first, passed, as one of well—"Maybe it's so and maybe it ain't—don't know."

In the next, we find that thought, study, the care, to understand why the anxiousness regarding the mother's influence in the life, concerning the other ones closer to the individual.

In the other, that projection of the necessity of some immediate action to save from some destructive forces, yet a channel, a means, as it were, projected with same.

"(Q) There is cause and effect in one of the fourth dimension; thus, the ability of the spirit entity, Pauline [...], to convey the message to [900]. In the fourth dimension, new events don't come to pass in time. Everything already is; thus, [137]'s ability to do what in the third dimension is called the future. Explain further the philosophical or metaphysical facts that these phenomena teach, that the mind of [900] may use this very condition that has come to his life and to the life of his dear ones around him, to better understand the great spirit force and its faculties and the laws governing thought transference, from the third dimension to the fourth dimension and vice versa.

"(A) These have all been given, in that as just given. Then study these, and making, see how the making of the application in the life of each becomes the phenomena of assistance. For truly is there found that the desire must precede the action and that directed thought becomes action in the concrete manner, through each force that the spiritual elements manifests through. And there then becomes the three manifestations in the three manners, in the three ways, all projections from a fourth dimensional condition into a third dimensional mind.

"(Q) Broaden your explanation or treatise now, using the above as an example, to meet the thoughts, studies and meditations of the enquiring mind of [900].

"(A) These may be broadened to many treatises. Sufficient that this should be first comprehended and understood in their elemental phases of projection in the three manners. Then, as these broaden in the mental mind, the ability to comprehend the greater scope of fourth dimensional conditions may come to the mind of [900].

"We are through for the present. (106-9)

Here's another reading related to dreams:

"(Q) What is the significance of dream I had Sat. night, regarding some big fine green beans on the sidewalk. Sam Ungerleider asked me to get a bag to put some in to take home. I went and tried everywhere, finally got a bag and saw Mr. Tompers, Jonas' partner, who said: "Take this name and this man will help you with Asheville factory."

"(A) In dreams, visions and experiences, each individual soul passes through or reviews or sees as from a different attitude those experiences of its own activities. And these are, in dreams or visions, as emblematical conditions in the experience of that soul-entity. At others we may find the activity of the body-physical regarding the diet or the activities in any experience of the mental body.

"This, as we find, is rather the vision, indicating the reviewing of the body-mind and its associations in and through the material things that it is passing in the present. This indicates first the activity in which the body has been in its body-mind trained or active in. The changing with individuals as the associations that may come about, but require that the activities of self be put into motion to profit through those associations, and in a manner that is as a container is indicated necessary to be found by the body. The associations in the bank and with the factory, that as of how through these varied activities there may come about the associations leading to that in that direction of activity.

"Then, this is as an emblematical condition of the experiences through which the body-mind is passing in the present.

"In making the application of same, then, these must be— as seen in the dream—sought out by self. One leading in a natural step from one to the other. As to what is to be accomplished, that self will not be bound save as in a manner that gives the body-mind and the whole of the entity's activity to act as it is inclined through the associations. (257-136)

The following is another reading about dreams and dreaming (I left it in its original file format):

TEXT OF READING 136-27 F 21 (Housewife)

This psychic reading given by Edgar Cayce at his office, 115 West 35th Street, Virginia Beach, Va., this 5th day of January, 1926, in accordance with request made by her husband, [900].

PRESENT

Edgar Cayce; Mrs. Cayce, Conductor; Gladys Davis, Steno.

READING

Time of Reading 10:40 A. M. Eastern Standard Time. New York City.

1. GC: You will have before you the body and the enquiring mind of [136] of New York City, and the dreams this body had on the dates which I will give you. You will give the interpretation and lesson to be gained from each of these, as I read same to you, and you will answer the questions I ask you regarding same.

2. EC: Yes, we have the body here. We have had this before, [136], with the dreams that have come from time to time. The dreams, we find, have come to this entity for that development, as has been given, in the body-mind of same. Ready for dream.

3. (Q) Wednesday morning, December 16, 1925. "I was to a house party with many others. One bus—the morning bus seemed to drive right up to the house, another, the one leading away, left from way below the cliff on which the house was located. Jagged stones, in step form led down to this outgoing bus. I decided suddenly to go home—I wanted to go home badly, so I rushed out and jumped off the cliff, catching myself one-half way down the stone steps. I made the bus, got on and was glad to be going home. I noticed S. and a whole

crowd of college girls in the other bus, up next to the house, climb in noisily—all clamoring."

(A) In this as is seen there are lessons being gained by the entity, as is seen in the recognition of all as college girls. The house party presents or represents that a special station, state or stop, as it were, in the education or development of the mental forces, is to take place in the mind. This is then presented in a manner as to how the entity would reach this conclusion towards going home, taking a sudden leap into that place where there has seemed to be before one of jagged stones, rocks, one of conditions hard to be understood by the entity. Yet, seemingly, it is the only mode, way or manner in which the entity may gain that portal that is desired in self. The seeing of others that make much noise is as but the clamor to the mental forces of entity from others that know the entity has embraced such a position or condition in its mental forces. It is a presentation, then, of conditions to arise in the life and mind, or mind of the entity becoming or being made a portion of the life. It refers, then, to the mental attitude of the entity toward conditions that had apparently been obnoxious, see?

4. (Q) "Ma was showing someone our house—the parlor, then the bedroom."

(A) This presents the coming to the entity of someone that would occupy these places.

5. (Q) Have these conditions already occurred?

(A) Already occurred.

6. (Q) Thursday night, December 17. "Heard [900] say 'Goodbye!'"

(A) This is the presentation of that condition in the mind of the entity through the subconscious forces of conditions that mean, as it means to the body-mind, "goodbye" from the entity. This has also happened in the life, see?

7. (Q) "Saw 4 aces and numbers in between, as follows:

2 3 4 ACE 2 ACE 3 ACE 4 ACE 2 3 4

(A) This is the presentation to the entity of that force exercised in numbers, and will be presented again in a different form for the entity's consideration. As is seen, One is the center, or the One Force. Two is that multiple of same with the division. Three is the force that is magnified in One—Two—see? with the One always giving the force, the power, or the magnified force of the number. Four is the half, or the double unit of Two, with its weaknesses, with those conditions as have been presented in numbers; yet the One showing, as always, the central force of strength, power or union.

8. (Q) Monday night, December 19. "Out loud so [900] heard: 'No, [900]—I'm fifty-one, not eighteen—you've got me as 18—I'm not that—I'm 51.'"

(A) This again is the presentation of the numbers five, one—six—one, eight—nine, see? and not as the nine the sufficient, the ending, the whole, as it were, of all forces as combined in the unit of numbers, but as the six, the multiple of the three unit in its action, and the entity SEES self—as the six; not as nine. That is, not as stable within self as the nine should imply.

9. (Q) Tuesday night, December 22. "Dreamed my Aunt H. bought a pair of black shoes and paid $95.00 for them." [This was 1926, so that would have been a ridiculous price for a pair of shoes!]

(A) The unreasonableness to the mind of the transaction, the unreasonableness of conditions which are to be existent in the life of the entity from that same reasoning standpoint. Lesson: Make a spiritual application of same, rather than material. Meaning, then, as of old: The usage of that necessary for the better development of self in any price is equal to that given out. For to obtain, that must be given that would be obtained."

As can see dreams are subconscious activities over outer life situations and circumstances. They can foreshadow upcoming events, deal with current events, and even review past events if there is some understanding to be gained. Adding a dream life to our physical life is a most helpful way to expand our consciousness and become of inner processes and perceptions that the outer rarely gets on its own.

Meditation
—"Magic Silence" Meditation—

Meditation is an altered state of consciousness. It is not a method for getting our normal consciousness to feel better. "You don't have the meditation because ... you want to feel better, but to attune self to the infinite!" (1861-18) We must set our normal, everyday selves aside and allow our deeper, spiritual selves to attune to the Infinite. This is perhaps the most fundamental and yet the most difficult requirement of meditation. But it can be done. The body, mind and soul are interconnected in such a way that certain actions will automatically lead to "the magic silence" and the awakening of our better selves.

There are actions that lead inward. We have two nervous systems. One (the Central Nervous System) we use mostly for our outer life and consciously functioning in the physical. The other (the Autonomic) governs those functions such as breathing and digestion that are taken care of without our conscious participation. What do these two nervous systems have to do with successful meditation? When we quiet the outer system and do something to stimulate the inner system, we are setting aside our outer selves and actually activating our souls. For example, let's sit down and stop using our musculoskeletal systems. Let's reduce our sense-perception by closing down our five senses — close our eyes, stop touching, listening, smelling and tasting. This quiets the outer system and the outer self. Now, let's take hold of some part of the inner system that the soul has charge of and let's alter it. The most popular one is the breath. The autonomic system, under the control of the subconscious mind and soul, is in charge of and directly connected to the breath. If we start changing the breath, we cause the soul and subconscious mind to become alert to the changes. This is an action that leads from our outer selves to our inner selves, and ultimately to an altered state of consciousness.

There are physical changes during meditation. Today we know from the research done in the '70s with transcendental meditators and others that the body goes through many changes during meditation. As researchers Wallace and Benson discovered, meditation causes measurable physical changes. "There is a reduction in oxygen consumption, carbon dioxide elimination and the rate and volume of respiration; a slight increase in the acidity of the arterial blood; a marked decrease in the blood-lactate level; a slowing of the heartbeat; a considerable increase in skin resistance; and an electroencephalogram pattern of intensification of slow alpha waves with occasional theta-wave activity" (Wallace & Benson, 1973, p. 266).

Reading 5752-3 expands on the wonderful changes: "Meditate ... in the inner secrets of the consciousness, and the cells in the body become aware of the awakening of the life...." The cells of the body become aware? According to the readings, every cell in the body has consciousness, and that consciousness may be raised or lowered. The reading goes on, "In the mind, the cells of the mind become aware of the life in the spirit." The cells of the mind, life in the spirit? Interesting concepts, aren't they? "God is Spirit, and those who worship Him must do so in spirit...." Then, if raising the consciousness leads to awareness of "life in the spirit," it leads to life with God — the Great Spirit. The wonderful thing about this whole process is that we activate it by entering into the magic silence.

For those of you who are just beginning with meditation or who have always had trouble meditating, let me spend a moment to describe this very simple yet effective way to meditate. Then, as you progress with your practice and develop your skills, you can move on to deep methods of meditation such as Kundalini meditation and Passage-In-Consciousness. The Magic Silence method is a simple yet powerful way for anyone to get into meditation — especially beginners and those who have difficulty meditating.

Using a combination of an affirmation and a mantra, coordinated with our breathing, we can enter into the magic silence. Let's use a modification of a line from Psalm 46, "Be still and know God." In order to fully succeed with this affirmation/mantra, not only do we need the power of the words, we must also take hold of the breath and create a breathing pattern that arouses the soul. It works like this: "Be STILL" [inhale slowly while feeling the word "still" and then exhale slowly] "and "Know GOD" [inhale slowly while feeling the word "God" and then exhale slowly]. Once you begin to "feel" the reality of these word "Still" and "God", let the breath go on automatic and abide in the feeling. If anything distracts you or feel you want to go deeper into the words, then repeat the deep inhalation and exhalation while saying the phrases. Keep the breath relaxed yet under your control.

If you are in the "stillness" or the "Godliness" between the phrases, remain in it as long as your consciousness holds there, breathing gently and evenly. If your consciousness wanders, then bring it back by saying (in your mind) one of the phrases and re-engaging the deep inhalation and exhalation cycle.

The more important parts of this practice the silent periods while feeling the power of essence of these words and their meaning. The phrases gather and direct the consciousness, and the spaces of silence are golden, or as the readings say, "magical." (137-3) So, as long as you are silent and still, stay there; don't feel a need to move on to the next phrase or to continue repeating the phrases. Abide in the powerful stillness and godliness.

This method of combining an affirmation/mantra with breathing will bring even the weakest meditator into a deep stillness and a heightened sense of Godliness.

To move deeper, add three "OM's" on the end of the last phrase: "Be STILL [feel and breathe], and know GOD [feel and breathe], OOOMMMM [feel and breathe] OOOMMMM [feel and breathe] OOOMMMM [feel and breathe]. This can be out loud in the beginning and then‡ silently in your mind as you go deeper. When chanting the OM incantation aloud, remember that true chanting is an inner sounding, not an outer singing. Keep the sound resonating within the cavities of your body. Beginning with the abdominal cavity, rising to the pulmonary cavity and then on into the cranial cavity, let the sound carry you deeper.

I've taught this method to people who have never meditated before, had them in a deep silence for twenty minutes, and watched them coming out of it with that wonderful glaze in their eyes that results from an altered state. Their outer self is moved yet uncertain as to exactly what has happened. But they know they have just meditated well. I've also had people who had tried meditation for years with little success come out of one of these sessions with the biggest smiles on their faces – victory at last!

The keys to succeeding with this method are three: First, the power of the words "still" and "God," and their effect on us. Second, the connection between the breath and the soul — allowing us to arouse our souls by taking hold of the breathing pattern. Third, the spaces of silence between the words while breathing. These spaces grow longer and longer as one practices. Eventually, an hour's meditation is easy (and recommended in the readings). According to the readings, and many other sources, the silence is in itself transforming. One need not "do" or "hear" anything when in meditation. Abide in the silence and it works its magic.

Now I would like us to look at another area of the total meditation picture. I would not recommend going on to this next practice (kundalini meditation) until you have practiced the Magic Silence method with much success, and feel you are ready to go deeper. As with medicine so it is with meditation: one person's poison may be another's cure, and activities that may be harmful at one stage in life may be quite helpful at another. You have to judge what is best for you now, and continue to evaluate your readiness as you progress.

It may appear contradictory to say that silence is in itself transforming and then to describe another form of meditation in which inner activities are used to affect greater transformation, but such is the case with the Cayce readings, and other sources. The explanation for this is that the manifold nature of full enlightenment and transformation is such that contradiction and paradox are elements of any method. After all, we are dealing with celestial beings in terrestrial forms, spirits in flesh, godlings of the Infinite God who are also human, and eternal beings living a temporary life. Paradox and contradiction are bound to be a part of any process that attempts to resolve or integrate these.

Furthermore, as we progress with our development, we naturally become more able to handle complexity and intricacy. We become more aware of and participate in the many aspects of the Godhead, the Universal Consciousness, with all its diversity.

—Kundalini (Energy) Meditation—

The life force is often symbolized as a raised serpent. Raising the serpent: not only Adam and Eve fell in the Garden, the serpent fell also. And, as Moses raised the serpent in the desert, so must we all raise the life force within us in order to receive the presence and the power of the Life Forces. One of the practices for doing this is kundalini meditation.

Like the Magic Silence method, this method will use words, breath and spaces of silence, but in more powerful ways. Since there is more power involved, there are more warnings in the readings about using this method without proper preparation and self-examination.

Cayce gave this warning: "But make haste SLOWLY! Prepare the body, prepare the mind, before ye attempt to loosen it in such measures or manners that it may be taken hold upon by those influences which constantly seek expressions of self rather than of a living, constructive influence of a CRUCIFIED Savior. Then, crucify desire in self; that ye may be awakened to the real abilities of helpfulness that lie within thy grasp. ...without preparation, desires of EVERY nature may become so accentuated as to destroy...." Therefore, let's examine our purposes, searching our hearts for our true passion. Is it cooperation and coordination with God, or are we still longing to gratify some lingering desires of our own self interests?

The Taoist meditators of *The Secret of the Golden Flower* (translated by Richard Wilhelm and commentated by Dr. Carl Jung) talk about the right method being like one wing of a bird, the other wing being the right heart. A wise seeker must remember, the bird cannot fly with only one wing. All seekers must have the right method *and* the right heart.

Setting our ideal or standard is the first step. The right-heart concept leads us naturally to the readings' teaching that an ideal should be raised as we seek to awaken the life force. What is our ideal? To whom or what do we look for examples of better behavior, better choices, better uses for our energies, better relating skills with others? What standard guides us in conceiving our better selves? Who is the author of our "Book of Life"? Is it the circumstances of life? Is it our self-interests?

These are important questions from the perspective of the Cayce readings, questions that should be considered before going on with the powerful kundalini forces aroused in this method of meditation. As the readings say, we can build a Frankenstein or a god using basically the same meditative method. It all depends on the ideal held as the practice progresses.

"FIND that which is to YOURSELF the more certain way to your consciousness of PURIFYING body and mind, before ye attempt to enter into the meditation as to raise the image of that through which ye are seeking to know the will or the activity of the Creative Forces; for ye are RAISING in meditation actual CREATION taking place within the inner self!"

The readings would advise anyone who feels unable to "set the carnal aside" and attune to a high ideal for the period of meditation to not meditate – and instead to pray. If the pray then changes you and you feel that you can set the carnal forces aside, you may enter into meditation. Otherwise, stay away from it. Meditation gives power to whatever is in the consciousness and desires of the person. Make sure these are pure and of the highest.

The Cayce readings present Jesus Christ as not only a high ideal but as a powerful force of protection for anyone seeking to loosen their life force, to open the bio-spiritual seals, and enter into the presence of God. Christ is presented as an advocate for us before the Godhead. To call on this protection and guidance is to call on the greatest resource available. However, the readings do not put the religion that formed around Jesus Christ above other religions. The readings are too universal for that. Seekers from any religious faith can use the power of Christ in their meditative practice and still remain loyal to their religion. Here's an example of this perspective, from reading 281-13:

"If there has been set the mark (mark meaning here the image that is raised by the individual in its imaginative and impulse force) such that it takes the form of the ideal the individual is holding as its standard to be raised to, ...then the individual (or the image) bears the mark of the Lamb, or the Christ, or the Holy One, or the Son, or any of the names we may have given to that which enables the individual to enter THROUGH IT into the very presence of that which is the creative force from within itself – see?...

Raising then in the inner self that image of the Christ, love of God-Consciousness, is making the body so cleansed as to be barred against all powers that would in any manner hinder."

Notice how "Christ" is given as equivalent to the "love of God-Consciousness." Seekers from any religion may have love of God-Consciousness. Christ in this perspective is more universal than the religion that possesses that name. Notice also how "love of God-Consciousness" cleanses us of self-interests that may hinder or harm us.

However, there is much more to this reading than ecumenism and protection. Cayce is giving us a great insight into just how a meditator may be transported from a good meditative stillness into the very presence of the Creative Force, God – with all the ramifications of such an experience. If in our imaginative forces we can conceive or form the ideal (the standard) to which we seek to be raised, then we (as the Revelation states) bear the mark or the sign of that power (whatever name we give it) that enables us to enter through it into the very presence of God within us, the Creative Force within us. Despite the power of some of the other techniques in this form of meditation, imaging the ideal is seminal to transformation. Reading 1458-1 points out our only limitation: "The entity is only limited to that it sets as its ideal." We are "gods in the making" if we can conceive ourselves to be such – in cooperation and coordination with the Great God.

This kundalini or life force is within the human body, the temple. Normally it is used in ways that dissipate it, eventually leading to aging and death of the body. All people are allowed to use their life force as they choose (at least within the parameters of their karma). Whether they dissipate it consciously or unconsciously makes no difference. When it's gone, it's gone. But it doesn't have to be this way. As the readings put it, "...if there will be gained that consciousness, there need not be ever the necessity of a physical organism aging ... seeing this, feeling this, knowing this, ye will find that not only does the body become revivified, but by the creating in every atom of its being the knowledge of the activity of this Creative Force ... spirit, mind, body [are] renewed."

The "elan vital" of the Western world and the "kundalini" of the Eastern world follows natural laws, and can be made to flow in rejuvenative ways that enhance and extend the life. This is not only possible with kundalini meditation, but it is a valuable goal to pursue. Here's one reading's statement on this: "How is the way shown by the Master? What is the promise in Him? The last to be overcome is death. Death of what? The soul cannot die, for it is of God. The body may be revivified, rejuvenated. And it is to that end it may, the body, transcend the earth and its influence." This meditation practice works directly with the forces of life.

Since this method uses the chakras and endocrine glands, we need a little device for awakening these spiritual centers within our bodies. Cayce us the secret words that he said Jesus taught to the holy women and disciples in the prayer he gave, known as the Lord's Prayer. Assuming that our ideals, purposes and hearts are in the right place, that we have crucified our selfish desires, conceived of our ideal, and drawn on the power and protection of the Christ, "love of God-Consciousness" – let's begin with these prayer-words for the seven chakras. These words vary with different practices, but the Cayce readings teach that one reason the Master created the Lord's Prayer was for this purpose. The readings give a slightly different version of the prayer, which we'll use. The readings are also comfortable with the feminine aspect of the Godhead as well as the masculine, so let's also use this. As you say the prayer, feel the meaning of the words as your consciousness is directed to the location of the chakra.

—Chart of Key Words in Lord's Prayer—

Key Word   Spiritual Center

Our Father who art in HEAVEN

                Third Eye - Pituitary - 7th

Hallowed be thy NAME

                Crown - Pineal - 6th

Thy kingdom come. Thy WILL

                Throat - Thyroid -5th

be done, as it is in Heaven, so on Earth. Give us this day our daily BREAD.

                Root - Gonads - 1st

And forgive us our DEBTS

                Solar Plexus - Adrenals - 3rd

as we forgive our debtors.

And lead us not into TEMPTATION

                Navel - Cells of Leydig - 2nd

but deliver us from EVIL

                Heart - Thymus - 4th

Some practitioners of this prayer-to-centers method add the following:

For Thine is the KINGDOM

                Throat - Thyroid - 5th

and the POWER

                Crown - Pineal - 6th

and the GLORY   Third Eye - Pituitary - 7th

forever.

To fully realize the power of this prayer, one must understand that it is intended to call forth the highest in each chakra. Just as we felt the words "stillness" and "God" in the earlier affirmation/mantra, so now we must feel or imagine the change brought on by these words and their meanings. Take your time. Consider this as part of the meditation period.

The order of the chakra prayer is significant in that it attempts to awaken the higher chakras before awakening the lower ones. This is the best approach. Awakening the first chakra before the seventh and sixth is like opening the serpent basket without the charm of the flute. The serpent is loose to its own interests, rather than under the charm of the higher music. Keep a higher ideal, a higher purpose, a right heart, and the consciousness focused predominantly on the higher centers. Draw the kundalini upward.

Now once again we take hold of the breath. This time we take a stronger hold and use it in ways that arouse the life force and draw it up through the chakras of this wonderful bio-spiritual instrument in which we abide – the human body. Why the breath? "BREATH is the basis of the living organism's activity. ...this opening of the centers or the raising of the life force may be brought about by certain characters of breathing – for, as indicated, the breath is power in itself; and this power may be directed...."

There are several breathing patterns we may use. The first is described often in the readings. It begins with a deep inhalation through the right nostril, filling the lungs and feeling strength! Then exhale through the mouth. This should be felt throughout the torso of the body – STRENGTH! After three of these, shift to inhaling through the left nostril and exhaling through the right (not through the mouth). This time feel the opening of your centers. As you do this left-right nostril breathing, keep your focus on the third eye and crown chakra, letting the other centers open toward these two. This will not be difficult because the sixth and seventh centers have a natural magnetism – just as the snake charmer's music.

When you have finished this breathing pattern, go through the prayer again slowly, directing your attention to each chakra as you recite the phrase and key word.

Then, begin the second breathing pattern. It goes like this. Breathe through your nostrils in a normal manner; however, with each inhalation feel or imagine the life force being drawn up from the lower parts of the torso to the crown of the head and over into the third-eye center. Hold the breath slightly, and then as you exhale, feel or imagine the life force bathing the chakras as it descends through them to the lowest center. Pause, then inhale while again feeling or imagining the drawing upward. Repeat this cycle at a comfortable pace – using your consciousness and breath to direct the movement in synchronization with the inhalations and exhalations. As the breath and life force rise, feel or imagine how they are cleansed and purified in the higher chakras. As they descend, feel how they bathe the chakras with this purified energy. Take your time; again, consider this as part of the meditation. Do about seven cycles of inhalations and exhalations.

"These exercises [yoga breathing] are excellent.... Thus an entity puts itself, through such an activity [yoga breathing], into association or in conjunction with all it has EVER been or may be. For it loosens the physical consciousness to the universal conscious-ness.... Thus ye may constructively use that ability of spiritual attunement, which is the birthright of each soul; ye may use it as a helpful influence in thy experiences in the earth."

After this breathing exercise it is a good time to use a rising incantation. Here's one from an ancient Egyptian mystical practice described in the readings. Breathe in deeply, then as you very slowly exhale, direct your consciousness to the lowest chakra and begin moving the life force upward as you chant in a drone "ah ah ah ah ah, a a a a a, e e e e e, i i i i i, o o o o o, u u u u u, m m m m m." Each sound is associated with a chakra. "Ah" with the root chakra (reading 2072-10, "this is not R, but Ah," as the "a" in spa). "A" with the lyden center (sounds like long "a" in able). "E" with the solar plexus (sounds like long "e" in eve). "I" with the heart (a long "i", as in high). "O" with the throat (long "o" as in open). "U" with the pineal (sounds like the "u" in true) . And, "m" with the third eye (like humming the "m" in room).

Remember that true incanting or chanting is an inner sounding which vibrates, stimulates and lifts the life force. It is done in a droning manner, with a monotonous, humming tone – vibrating the vocal cords and then directing this vibration to the chakras, thus vibrating them. Feel the chakras being tuned to the specific sound/vibration, and then carry your consciousness upward as the sound changes. Do this chanting three or more times, or until you feel its effect. You may also want to finish this chanting portion of the practice with a few soundings of the great OM chant (as in home).

Often at this point in the meditation, the head will be drawn back, the forehead and crown may have pronounced sensations or vibrations, and the upper body and head may be moving back and forth, or side to side, or in a circular motion (circular is preferable). These are all natural results of the practice and are identified as such in the readings. In the Revelation, St. John associates body-shaking ("earthquakes") with the opening of the sixth chakra, followed by "silence in heaven" as the seventh chakra opens.

Now we want to move from bodily enhancements into our mind and higher consciousness, so let the breathing and body go on autopilot.

At this point in the practice, the whole of the body, mind and soul are aroused and alert. Now, the ideal held is the formative influence, and development proceeds according to the ideal held.

The mind has a somewhat different experience in this type of meditation than it does in the Magic Silence method. All self-initiated activity is suspended. The mind has been changing as we have raised the energies of the body. By now it is very still, yet quite alert. Stay here. Do not draw away or attempt to affect anything. Heightened expectancy and alertness is an excellent state of mind at this point. Here's

205

where we have the greatest opportunity to receive the Life Forces, or God. Completely open your consciousness to God's mind. We now reach a point in the meditation where we turn around from our constant outer-directed thought stream, to become one with God's consciousness, and purely receptive.

The readings say we should have a strong sense of expansion and universalization while in this state. They also recommend that we imagine expansion as we progress toward this place in the meditation. The imaginative forces should be used to help us reach higher consciousness. So, imagine expansion as you raise the life force in the early stages of the practice. According to the readings, the pineal's primary functioning is "the impulse or imaginative" force. It is the pineal chakra that aids in the transition from heightened material consciousness to real spiritual consciousness. Use your imaginative forces to aid in this transition. Also, reading 294-141 adds, "Keep the pineal gland operating and you won't grow old – you will always be young!" Again we see the rejuvenative powers of stimulating the imagination.

Reading 281-13 describes more of what occurs. "The spirit and the soul is within its encasement, or its temple within the body of the individual - see? With the arousing..., it rises along that which is known as the Appian Way, or the pineal center, to the base of the brain, that it may be disseminated to those centers that give activity to the whole of the mental and physical being. It rises then to the hidden eye in the center of the brain system, or is felt in the forefront of the head, or in the place just above the real face - or bridge of nose, see?"

As we have seen, the soul is encased in the second chakra of the body, the lyden center. From this chakra it is drawn upwards by the magnetism that results from stimulating the pineal center. It rises to the base of the brain and into the pineal center, the crown chakra. In ancient Egyptian mysticism, the lyden center is represented by the lower gate and pharaoh of the lower Nile, while the pineal center is the upper gate and pharaoh of the upper Nile. In *The Book of the Master of the Hidden Places* (more commonly titled *The Egyptian Book of the Dead*) there are ancient Egyptian pictures of a young man named "Ani" encouraging his soul to pass through the lower gate, and later Ani's soul is seen at the threshold of the upper gate, ready to make that wonderful passage into the higher consciousness. The caption under these pictures reads, "Hail ye gods who make souls to enter into their spiritual bodies. Grant ye that the soul of the reunited Ani, triumphant, may come forth before the gods, and that his soul may have peace in the Hidden Place."

The power gained from this type of meditation is not used to rule but to allow more of God's influence to come into our lives and into this dimension. Raising the Life Force within the body is key to higher consciousness and resurrecting mortal flesh as spiritualized flesh.

We are the channels of God in this realm, if we choose to be so. We could literally transform this realm if more of us developed ourselves to be better, clearer channels of the Life Force, the Great Spirit, God. The residual effect of this is that our individual lives become more fulfilling, abundant, rejuvenated and eternal.

From the readings' perspective, "In the doing comes the understanding" – not in the talking, the reading, the believing, the knowing, or thinking – but in the *doing*. So take up your practice. Not just to feel better but that the Infinite may manifest in our finite condition, lifting us to a more wonderful life!

—Humor—

From Cayce's perspective humor was human trait to be cultivated! He even saw it as being a lifesaver when troubles abound and turmoil casts its shadow over life. Here are some of his comments on humor:

"That this entity has a sense of humor has oft been a saving grace, in not only this experience but in others. And this brings about those abilities that are worth while, if they are applied in the present experience." (2788-1)

"One who is at all times inclined towards good humor, and might at times well be called a wit. At TIMES the entity sees so WELL the humor in SO MANY situations as to appear to see the ridiculous rather than that which is the creative force in humor. DO NOT lose this sense of humor; it will be a means for saving MANY an unseeming situation." (2421-2)

"The entity at times is dramatic in such expression. And this may be used or applied in the associations or activities with others. Then, these applications more in the form of mirth or comics should be stressed, rather than too much of dramatics. For, the entity is inclined at times to be moody, and self-condemning - and may speak that which may be a hindrance, unless the ridiculous or the comic or funny side of every problem is taken into consideration." (2655-1)

"One whose sense of humor has and will oft save many an unpleasant situation. Keep that humor! Rather cultivate same. Entertain it, and use it also in your abilities as a singer, as a teacher, as an announcer." (5262-1)

"One that finds a sense of humor in most every situation, and this is something that should be encouraged ever in the experience of the entity." (3205-1)

"It is well that the entity cultivate that of humor, or the funny side of an experience and not become morose, self-centered, nor to that extent as to only see the serious side of experiences, associations or the like. Cultivate reading comics, wit and humor, those stories or visualizations of activities that have the humor in same." (2648-1)

"The entity should attempt–seriously, prayerfully, spiritually–to see even that as might be called the ridiculous side of every question–the humor in same. Remember that a good laugh, an arousing even to what might in some be called hilariousness, is good for the body, physically, mentally, and gives the opportunity for greater mental and spiritual awakening.

"That seriousness with which the body (and mind) takes on the material as well as the mental and social relationships is not good. While the happenings, the experiences even in the material sojourn may have at times tended to convince the body of the seriousness of living, know that life should be joyous, happy, open, and ALL that brings hope.

"For, in the seriousness of it all, know that the very fact of consciousness itself, the very fact of an awareness of self and self's emotions, is an expression of the awareness within of the divine and of His (God's) hope for you. And if He be with you, what matters what others think or say—in the material world?" (2647-1)

"One that should cultivate more the humorous side of life; see some wit, some humor. Not that which is at the expense of another; that is, never laugh at anyone, but laugh WITH others often." (2327-1)

"(Q) How can a sense of humor in this body be developed or cultivated?

"(A) It is natural with the body. The deeper sense of humor is not always appreciated by those conditions as exist in the surroundings. But if there is the health ... this is a NATURAL DEVELOPMENT of the body." (773-13)

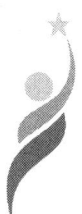

List of Illustrations

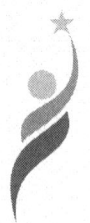

ILLUSTRATIONS

Central Nervous System

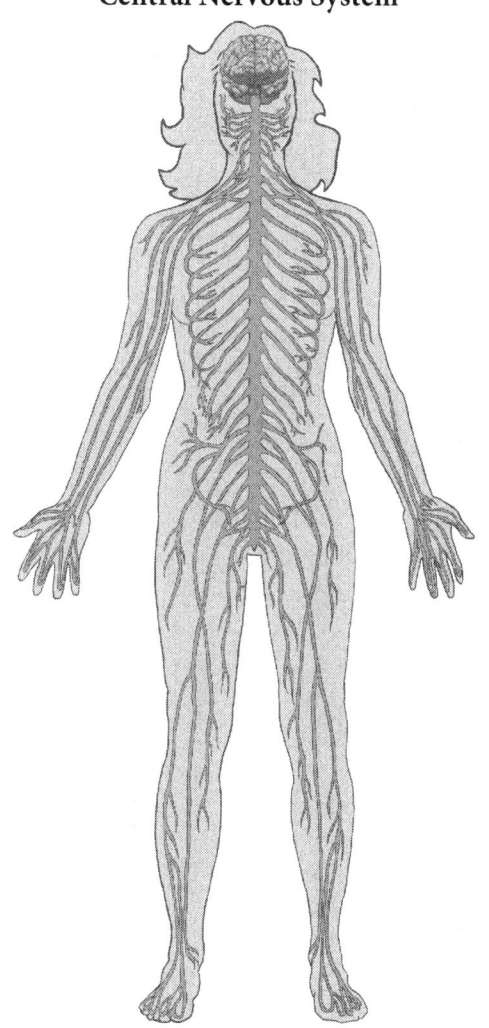

The central nervous system and the peripheral nervous system include the nerves in the brain and spinal cord, and all other nerves in the body are part of the peripheral nervous system. The Central System is safely contained within the skull and vertebral canal of the spine. (Source: ncbi.nim.nih.gov — National Center for Biotechnology Information)

Autonomic Nervous System
2 Parts: Sympathetic & Parasympathetic

Sympathetic System

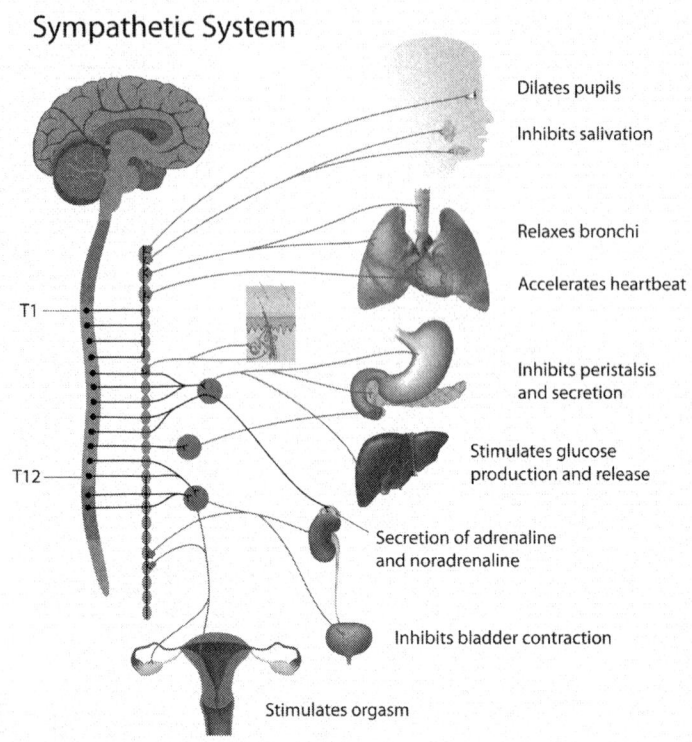

Dilates pupils

Inhibits salivation

Relaxes bronchi

Accelerates heartbeat

T1

Inhibits peristalsis
and secretion

Stimulates glucose
production and release

T12

Secretion of adrenaline
and noradrenaline

Inhibits bladder contraction

Stimulates orgasm

The sympathetic nervous system prepares the body for action. Some of its primary functions are to increase the heart rate and increase the release of sugar from the liver into the blood stream, dilate the bronchi to increase their diameter for more air, retain urine during activity, slow digestion so more energy for action is available, increase the pulse rate and heighten blood pressure levels for action, our pupils dilate, sharpening sight. It is also the remnant of our ancestor's need for the fast-reacting fight-or-flight activity when danger is imminent. Today this fast-reacting system engages during rush-hour traffic, arguments, missing appointments, and hurrying to get all that have to do in little to no time.

Parasympathetic System

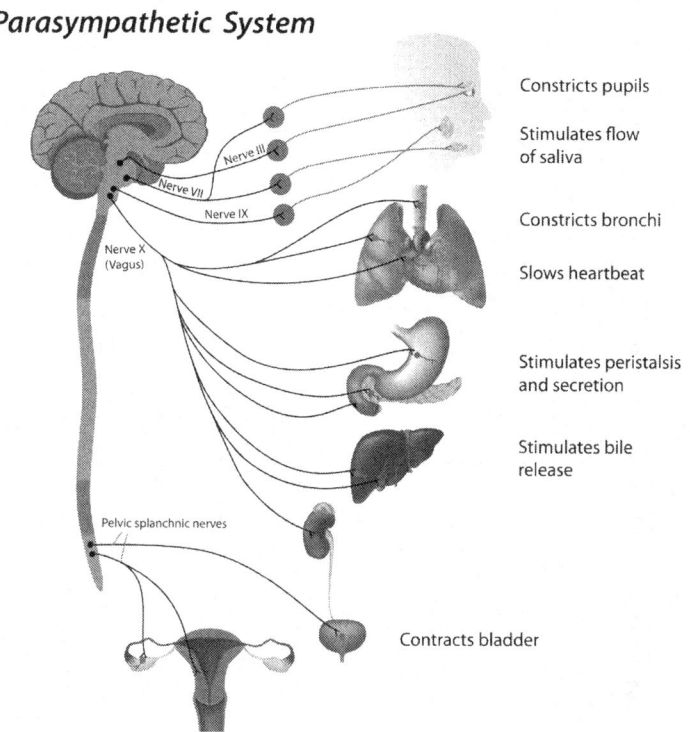

Constricts pupils

Stimulates flow
of saliva

Constricts bronchi

Slows heartbeat

Stimulates peristalsis
and secretion

Stimulates bile
release

Contracts bladder

Nerve III
Nerve VII
Nerve IX
Nerve X
(Vagus)
Pelvic splanchnic nerves

The parasympathetic nervous system activates tranquility and redirects functions to restore the body's homeostasis (balance and equilibrium internally), such as stimulating the secretion of saliva and digestive enzymes in the stomach for a rest-and-digest time, decrease the pulse rate and slow down the blood pressure, constrict the bronchi so breathing becomes more shallow and calm, stimulates urination and evacuation of contents in the rectum to reduce toxins in the body. This system makes adjustments to re-stabilize and renew the body. It plays an important role in stress reduction.

Circulation System for Blood

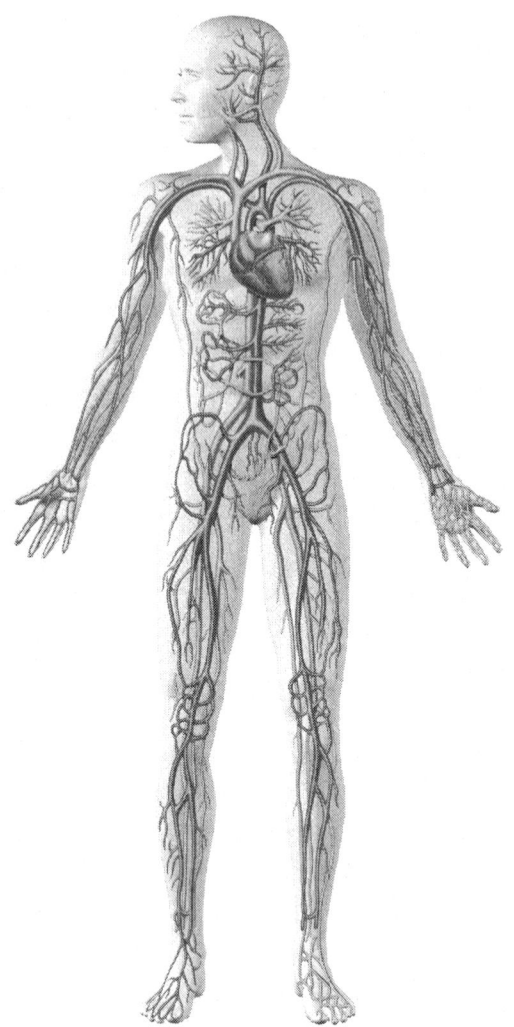

The heart pumps oxygenated and deoxygenated blood throughout the body in a complex system of arteries, veins, and capillaries.

Circulation System for Lymph

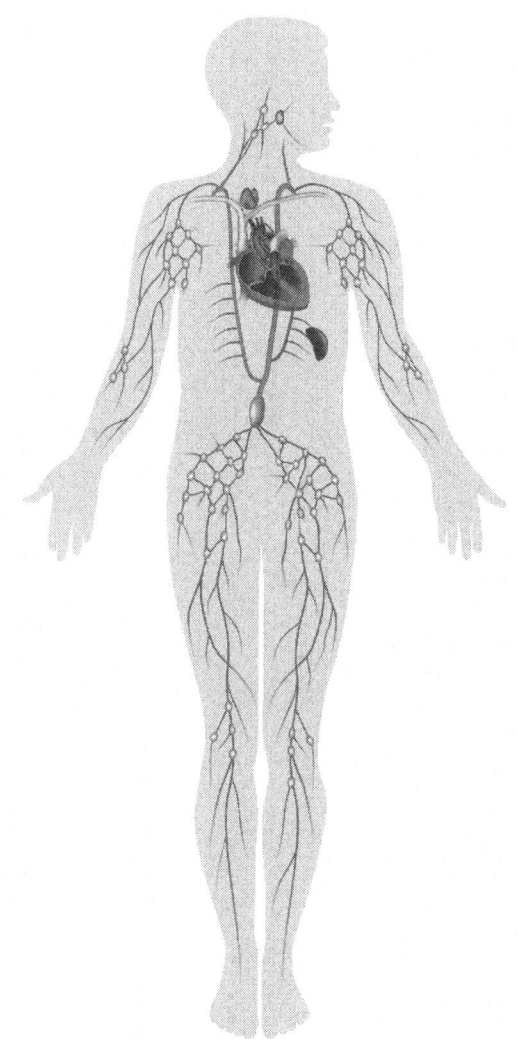

More on the lymph on the next page.

Lymph System Detail

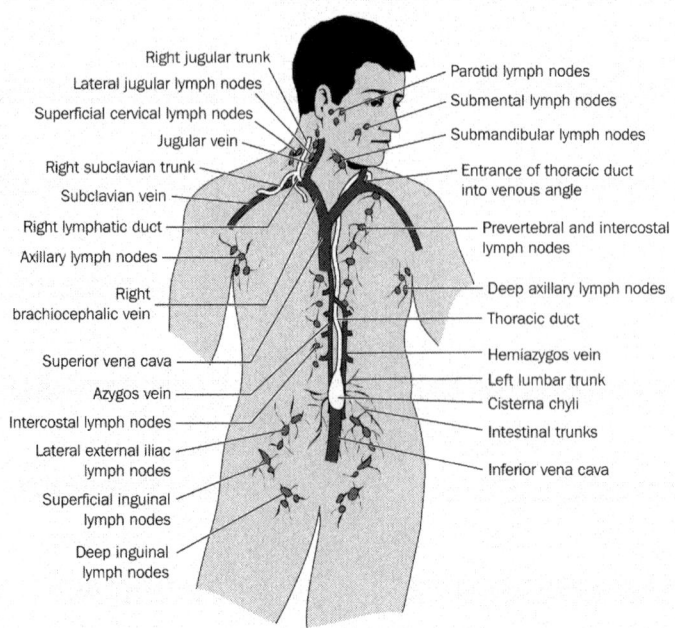

The lymphatic system is a network of tissues and organs that help rid the body of toxins, waste and other unwanted materials. The primary function of the lymphatic system is to transport lymph, a fluid containing infection-fighting white blood cells, throughout the body. (Source: livescience.com)

Endocrine Glandular System (Female)

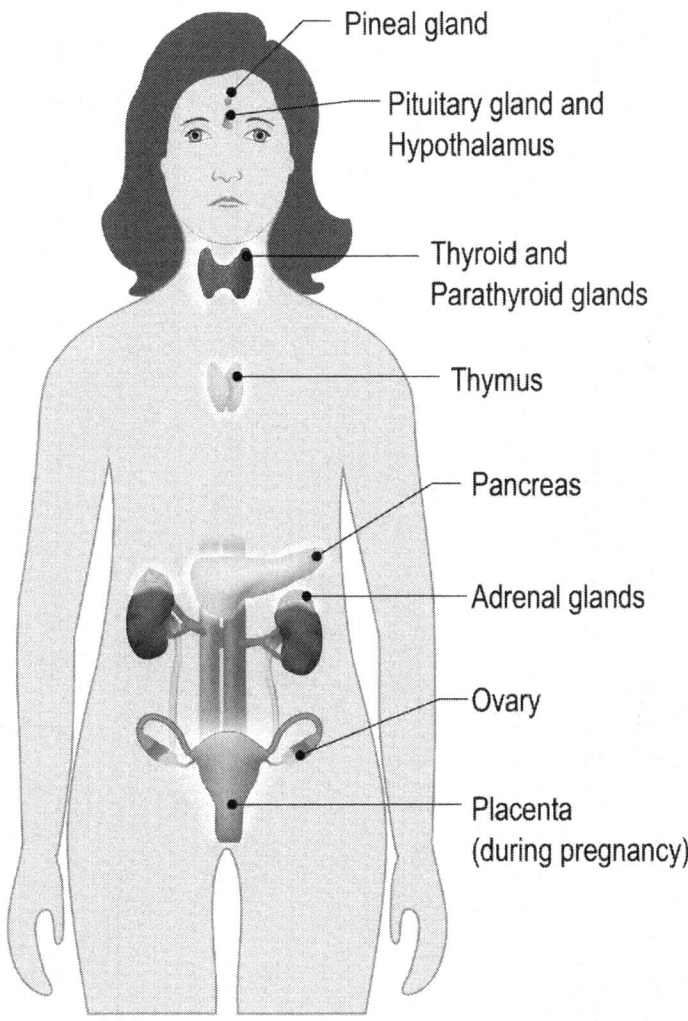

- Pineal gland
- Pituitary gland and Hypothalamus
- Thyroid and Parathyroid glands
- Thymus
- Pancreas
- Adrenal glands
- Ovary
- Placenta (during pregnancy)

The Cells of Leydig are missing in this diagram. They would be around the genitals and would correlate to the navel chakra.

Endocrine Glandular System (Male)

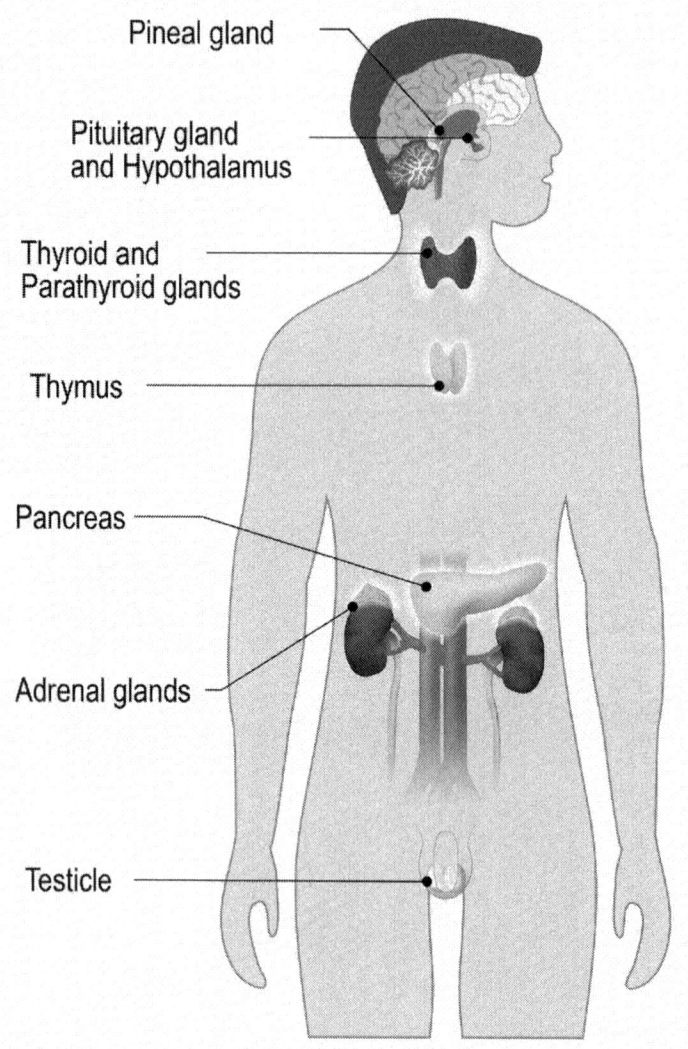

Pineal gland

Pituitary gland
and Hypothalamus

Thyroid and
Parathyroid glands

Thymus

Pancreas

Adrenal glands

Testicle

The Cells of Leydig are missing in this diagram. They would be around the genitals and would correlate to the navel chakra.

Spiritual Centers in the Human Body

The Life Force (Kundalini) flows through the body during meditation in the shape of a cobra in the striking position. That is why a raised cobra is the traditional symbol for bodily energy during meditation in ancient India, Egypt, and Mayan lands. It rises from lower chakras, up the spine to the base of the brain, and then to the center of the brain and over to the large frontal lobe of a human brain, finally to the master gland of the body: the pituitary.

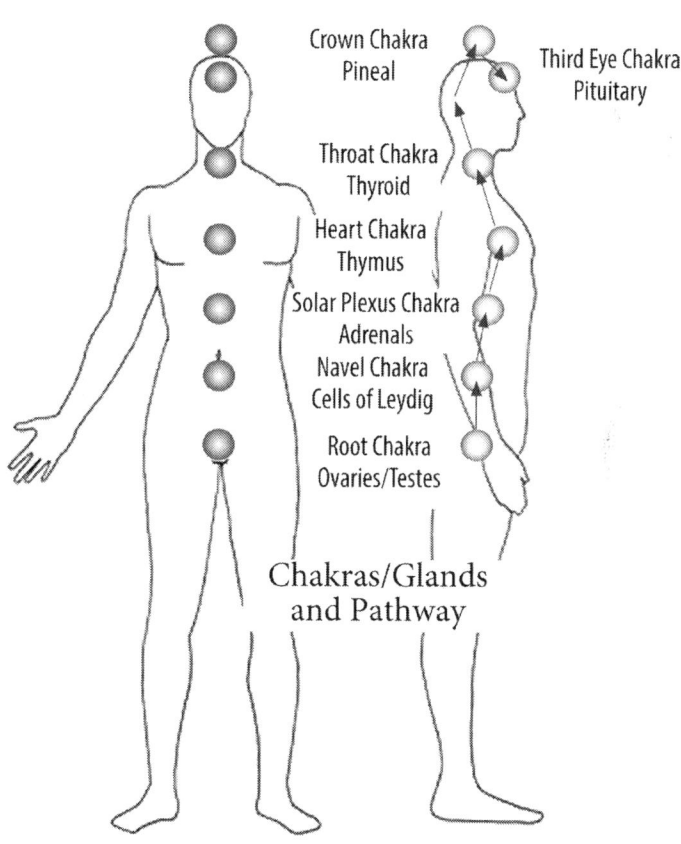

Crown Chakra
Pineal

Third Eye Chakra
Pituitary

Throat Chakra
Thyroid

Heart Chakra
Thymus

Solar Plexus Chakra
Adrenals

Navel Chakra
Cells of Leydig

Root Chakra
Ovaries/Testes

Chakras/Glands
and Pathway

Spinal Column

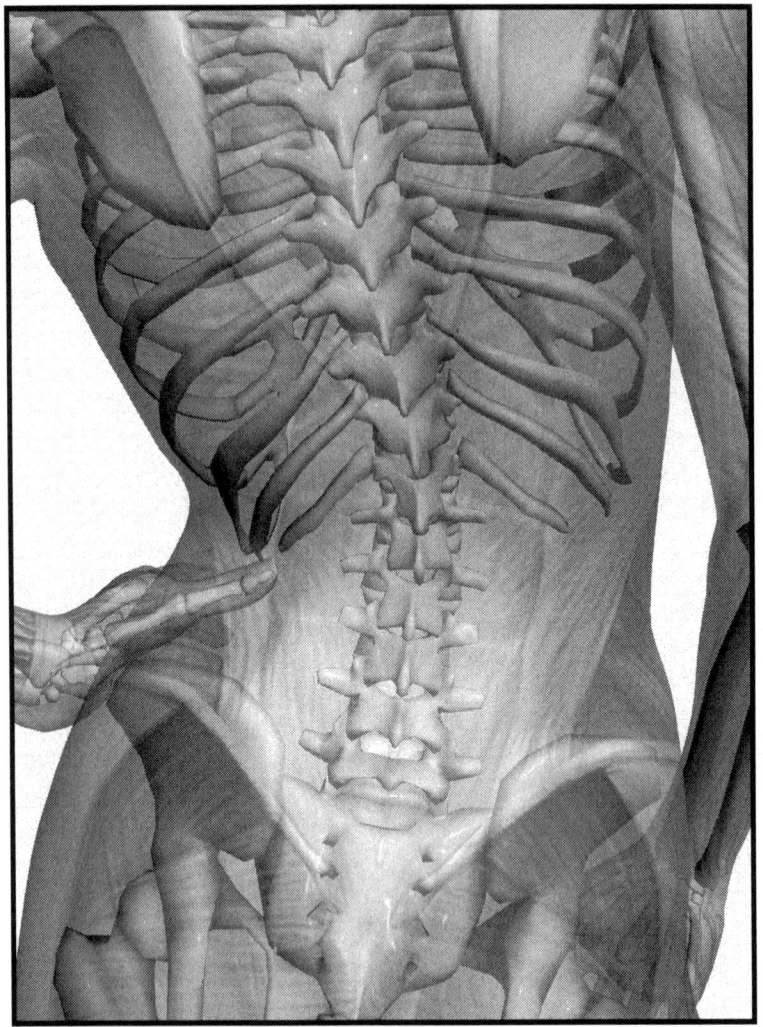

The human body is an amazing wonder of Life's creativity!

SPINAL CORD

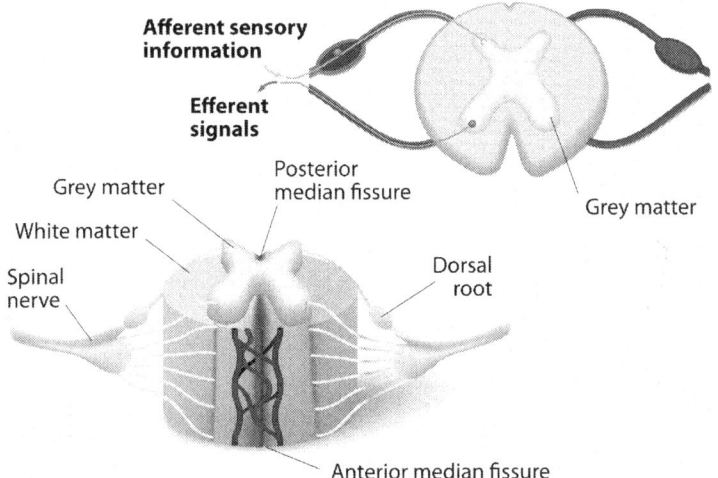

Afferent sensory information

Efferent signals

Grey matter

White matter

Spinal nerve

Posterior median fissure

Grey matter

Dorsal root

Anterior median fissure

Vertebrae Detail with Spinal Cord & Nerves

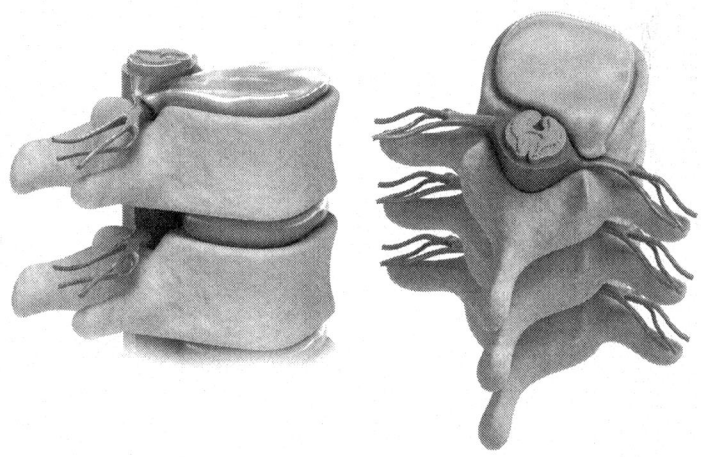

ANATOMY OF THE LARGE INTESTINE

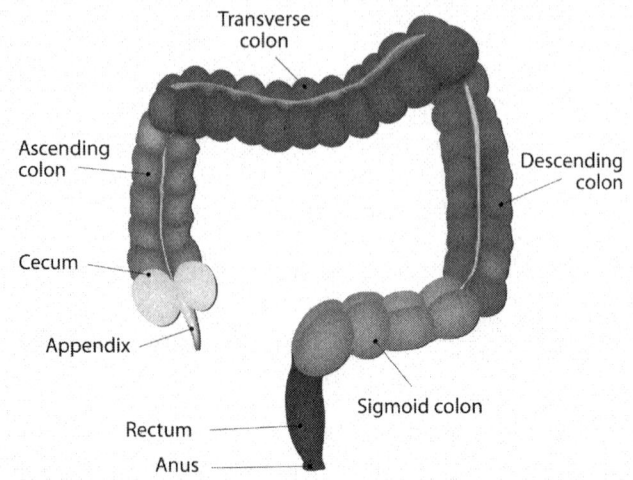

Thanks to improvements in prevention, early detection, and treatment, more than a million people in the US count themselves as survivors of colon or rectum cancer. A colonoscopy (koe-lun-OS-kuh-pee) is an exam used to detect changes or abnormalities in the large intestine (colon) and rectum. During a colonoscopy, a long, flexible tube is inserted into the rectum. A tiny video camera at the tip of the tube allows the doctor to view the inside of the entire colon. If necessary, precancerous polyps or other types of abnormal tissue can be removed through the scope during a colonoscopy. Tissue samples (biopsies) can be taken during a colonoscopy as well. (Source: Mayo Clinic.org)

Resources for Further Study & Assistance

Books:

The Edgar Cayce Handbook for Health Through Drugless Therapy by Harold Reilly and Ruth Hagy Brod

The Oil That Heals by William McGarey, M.D.

The Miracle Oil: Secrets of Edgar Cayce's Palma Christi Revealed by David E. Kukor

The Alkalizing Diet by Istvan Fazekas

Edgar Cayce's Quick & Easy Remedies: A Holistic Guide to Healing Packs, Poultices, and Other Homemade Remedies by Elaine Hruska, MA

Edgar Cayce's Massage, Hydrotherapy, and Healing Oils by Sandra Duggan, RN

Your Key to Good Health: Unlocking the Power of Your Lymphatic System by Elaine Hruska, MA

Once Cause, Many Ailments: The Leaky Gut Syndrome by John Pagano DC

Edgar Cayce on Healing Foods by William McGarey MD

Videos:

Edgar Cayce's Quick & Easy Remedies: A Holistic Guide to Healing Packs, Poultices, and Other Homemade Remedies by Elaine Hruska, MA (there is also a book and video combination offer from A.R.E. that saves money)

Edgar Cayce's Quick & Easy Home Remedies featuring J.P. Amonte DC and Renée Branch, CMT

Meditative Techniques to Boost Soul Growth by John Van Auken

The Akashic Record and the Illusion of Time by Kevin Todeschi

Discovering Your Soul's Mission by Mark Thurston Ph.D.

Reincarnation: The Story of Our Souls by John Van Auken

Tonics & Devices:

Baar.com is the official suppler of Edgar Cayce products and they have information on Cayce.com.

Baar Products, PO Box 60, Downingtown, PA 19335 USA

Orders: 1-800-269-2502 Customer Service: 1-610-873-4591

The Edgar Cayce Center

Association for Research & Enlightenment, Inc.
215 67th Street
Virginia Beach, VA 23451 USA
800-333-4499
757-428-3588
EdgarCayce.org
AREcatalog.com

Edgar Cayce Spa & Health Center
is located on the campus in Virginia Beach
Email: Spa@EdgarCayce.org

Cayce-Reilly School of Massage
Offers massage therapy certification programs, continuing
education workshops, and a student massage clinic. Includes
training in hydrotherapy and healing applications.
COMTA Certified
757-457-7270
Fax: 757-428-0398
info@caycereilly.edu

Atlantic University
is a fully accredited university
offering Master's Degree Programs
in Transpersonal Psychology through
"at-distance-education"
DETC Accredited
AtlanticUniv.edu
757-631-8101 or 800-428-1512
Fax 757-631-8096
It is headquartered on the A.R.E.
campus in Virginia Beach

INDEX

Other Books by John Van Auken

◆ *Passage in Consciousness: A Guide to Expanding Our Minds and Raising the Life Forces in Our Bodies through Deep Meditation*

◆ *Reincarnation & Karma: Our Soul's Past-Life Influences*

◆ *From Karma to Grace: The Power of the Fruits of the Spirit*

◆ *Edgar Cayce on the Spiritual Forces Within Us*

◆ *Edgar Cayce's Amazing Interpretation of The Revelation*

◆ *Hidden Teachings of Jesus*

◆ *A Broader View of Jesus Christ*

◆ *Edgar Cayce and the Kabbalah: A Resource for Soulful Living*

All Titles and more are available on Amazon.com, Createspace.com, AREcatalog.com, and JohnVanAuken.com

John Van Auken
Living in the Light Newsletter
P.O. Box 4942
Virginia Beach, VA 23454
JohnVanAuken.Newsletter@Gmail.com
JohnVanAuken.com

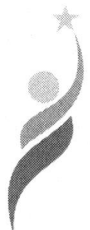

227

Printed in Great Britain
by Amazon